THE BIO-DIET

THE BIO-DIET

A doctor's plan to
eliminate hunger,
change your body chemistry,
lose weight—and keep it off!

LUIS A. GUERRA, M.D.

CROWN PUBLISHERS, INC.
NEW YORK

NOTE: Check with your doctor before starting this or any other diet plan.

Copyright © 1982 by Luis A. Guerra, M.D.
All rights reserved. No part of this book may be reproduced or utilized in any form or by any means, electronic or mechanical, including photocopying, recording, or by any information storage and retrieval system, without permission in writing from the publisher.

Inquiries should be addressed to Crown Publishers, Inc., One Park Avenue, New York, New York 10016

Printed in the United States of America
Published simultaneously in Canada by General Publishing Company Limited

Library of Congress Cataloging in Publication Data

Guerra, Luis A.
 The Bio-diet: A doctor's plan to eliminate hunger, change your body chemistry, lose weight—and keep it off!

 Includes index.
 1. Reducing diets. I. Title.
RM222.2.G78 1982   613.2'5   81-12524
ISBN: 0-517-545780   AACR2

10 9 8 7 6 5 4 3 2

*To Thelma, Claudia, Alejandro Luis,
Lyda, Mary,
and the memory of my father, Jose,
and my uncles, Luciano and Francisco*

Acknowledgments

I would like to thank Sandra Rivera and Kathy Naughton for their assistance and generous help on this project.

L.G.

Contents

Introduction, ix

1. Why You Eat, 1

Senses and the Appetite, 3; Taste and Sweetness, 5; Curbing a Sweet Tooth, 6; Women Are Different, 7; Rational Eating, 8; The Exercise Factor, 9; A Better Way to Relax, 9

2. What You Should Know Before Starting the Bio-Diet, 11

Composition of Foods, 13; What Happens When You Eat, 13; Natural Appetite Suppressants, 16; Using Your Body Chemistry to Your Advantage, 20; The Bio-Diet and Your Appetite, 21; Carbohydrates, 22; Soluble Fiber, 25; The Pattern of Intake, 28; The Good and Bad of Protein, 28; Fat Intake and Fat Deposits, 30; How to Prolong Morning Satiation, 35; Water Intake and Water Retention, 36; Eating Control Through "Natural Food Supplements," 37; It's Time to Diet, 38

3. The Bio-Diet, 39

The Bio-Diet: One Week Work, One Week Fun, 42; Bio-Diet Work Weeks, 43; Bio-Diet Break Weeks, 45; Diet Components, 46; Allowed Fluids, 47; Starter Vegetables, 49; Filler Vegetables, 50; Recommended Proteins, 51; Allowed Spices, Sauces, and Dressings, 52; Fruit Starters, 53; The No-Choice Bio-Diet, 54; Weekly Diets, 55

4. Questions I Have Been Asked by My Patients, 65

5. Exercise, 87

Recipe for Living Longer, 89; How Exercise Works, 89; How to Get Your Muscles to Burn More Calories, 91; Exercise a Lot . . . Diet a Little, 92; A Word for Women, 92; Losing and Regaining Weight (the Yo-Yo Syndrome), 95; Interval Training Is the Answer, 96; Training with Weights versus Weight Lifting, 97; The Exercise Prescription, 98; Total Reducing or Spot Reducing, 99; Warm-ups, 101; Interval Training: General Part, 104; Interval Training: Specific Part, 109; Special Situations, 121; Shoes and Leg Circulation, 124; Massage, Steam Baths, and Saunas, 124; Cellulite, 125; How to Stay Motivated to Exercise, 126

6. Relaxation Reflex, 127

How to Relax, 130; Desensitization, 131; Conditioned Reflex, 131; Relaxation, 132; How to Use the Tape, 133; The Tape, 134

Afterword, 139
Glossary, 141
Index, 143

Introduction

You have probably tried to lose weight by dieting, going to a gym, or changing your behavior. This book shows you the most simple, effective, and comprehensive solution to your fat problem. Unlike fad diet books, *The Bio-Diet* provides you with abundant scientific information that you can put to work for you!

Reducing diets used to be concerned with *what* you ate. The Bio-Diet will show you *when* and *how* to eat to change your body chemistry and stay slim.

Recent research has documented the interplay of food intake and body chemistry. By eating some types of food in a specified order, you can change your body chemistry to your advantage. Your body reacts to what you have eaten by changing the chemical composition of the organs that control your appetite and the distribution of fat.

Your body has natural appetite suppressants, appetite stimulants, and substances that burn fat. You can activate any one of these factors if you know what, when, and how to eat. The Bio-Diet is based on the latest scientific research and is designed to increase the natural appetite suppressants and substances that burn fat while decreasing the absorption of what you have eaten. The Bio-Diet will keep you satisfied while providing few calories and a lot of food. The Bio-Diet has the following objectives:

1. To activate natural appetite suppressants.
2. To avoid an increase in the substances that produce hunger.
3. To decrease food absorption.

But you must learn *about* you before *changing* you! You should know more about the malfunctioning of your overweight body, the importance of your mental attitude toward weight loss, why you eat, overeat, or eat the wrong things. The more you know, the more sense this program will make.

Like any program that changes your eating patterns, increases your muscle activity, and produces fat loss, the Bio-Diet should be started only after getting a complete physical examination and approval from your doctor. Your doctor should follow your progress to avoid any unforeseen, unwanted results.

Would you like to accomplish your weight goal and still eat many of the things you like? While following my diet, you "work" hard on a strict diet for one week, and then you have a "break" for a week during which you can eat starches and lots of fruit. You don't count calories.

To change your chemistry, you must change your food intake. On my diet, a small protein breakfast prolongs the natural overnight appetite suppression. At lunch, you eat foods that cut down the absorption of calories. Dinner ends the day with plenty of food intake and sets your chemistry for the next day. This is a healthy, tasty, varied, and balanced diet. You can follow it anywhere to obtain its benefits: at home, at a luncheonette, or at a fancy restaurant.

The Bio-Diet, based on new data including some from the Skylab program, will teach you how to attain your desired weight and become physically fit while exercising only 36 minutes a week.

Until recently it was impossible to specifically target fat loss. This is no longer true. I have prepared a program for localized fat loss based on my years of practice as a physician specializing in weight control. This means that unsightly thighs, excessive hips and buttocks, or bulging tummies can be slimmed without your becoming a skeleton from the waist up. You can also lose all over, if you so desire, by exercising more.

The exercises can be tailored to your specific problem. Skip the arm exercises if you are interested only in slimming your thighs, but do not concentrate on dieting while conveniently forgetting to exercise. Remember that all factors are related, so if you binge one day, offset your overeating by increasing the exercises for that day.

You will also learn to control the stress that often leads to overeating. You might wonder what stress control has to do with losing weight. Your emotions control your eating to a great degree. To control emotions such as anxiety, boredom, and depression, which trigger your appetite, you must learn some new skills. I teach my patients a procedure that they can use anywhere when confronted with tension. The technique is, in fact, a reflex much like the one that occurs when you jump at a sudden noise or close your eyes when a ball is coming toward your face. I call it "The Relaxation Reflex."

The Bio-Diet is based on life processes. It is centered on your body and the way your body works. At some point in your life, your body chemistry changed from that of slimness to one of overweight. It is now time to reverse the process! If you stay on the Bio-Diet for three months, you will change your body chemistry so you can lose weight and stay slim for the rest of your life.

NOTE. Check with your doctor before starting this or any other diet plan.

1
Why You Eat

Everything that happens to you can be traced back to a physiological reaction. Even emotional responses are chemical. Your lack of motivation for following a diet has physiological roots. Some diet books try to modify behavior, but my book will help you understand why it is the wrong chemistry that produces the wrong psychological response. It is all there in your body—I will help you learn what to do to change it.

The Bio-Diet will explain why you eat, what happens during digestion, why certain people have greater trouble losing weight than the general population, and how you can manipulate your body chemistry to lose weight and stay slim. Anything that is malfunctioning can be changed and returned to normal. You will learn to concentrate on those chemical actions rather than on calorie counting. It's very simple. Your appetite depends on the order of food intake, the composition of the foods, and the amount you eat. And you can control your appetite if you understand it.

Senses and the Appetite

Animals and human beings are attracted to pleasant things and are repelled by unpleasant ones. We might want to eat fresh-baked bread, but can easily refuse a rotten apple. Information about food is stored in our cells and guides our choices.

The odors, taste, and textures of food are perceived by your senses and checked against your stored genetic information, and then your appetite is triggered. Odor and texture do not indicate how many calories are in a food—unpleasant-smelling foods, such as certain cheeses, might have high calorie counts while some good-smelling foods, such as fresh oranges, are low in calories.

The sight and/or smell of food can start a biochemical reaction called appetite. Why do you feel hungry when you smell food? A researcher blew a series of attractive food odors at animals that had finished feeding. The food odors provoked a rapid revival of interest in food, and most of the animals started eating again. Odors influence what foods an animal will eat as well as how much food is consumed. This is also true in humans, for whom the sense of smell has a lot to do with the urge to eat. Food odors are signals of the pleasure to come from eating. Anticipation of that pleasure, elicited by the food odor, might be more important than the taste itself. You might derive more satisfaction from the smell than from the act of eating—things often don't live up to our expectations.

People who have an impaired olfactory sense frequently have poor appetites. You can use this fact to your advantage. For instance, if you smell a strong perfume before eating, it will mask your olfactory sense and you might feel more in control of your appetite.

The degree to which all of your senses are stimulated will affect your eating. The greater variety of flavor, odor, and color you are presented with, at a smorgasbord, for example, the more you will eat. This means you will overeat in certain situations even when you do not feel hungry.

Many overweight people have a poor sense of taste. They can't tell the difference between good ground steak and cheap hamburger meat with fillers. Poor taste capacity leads to decreased eating satisfaction, which often results in overeating. Mineral supplements containing extra zinc, copper, and nickel can improve this condition.

The sense of touch is also important in food intake. If you touch the lips and cheeks of a newborn, its mouth, head, and neck will respond. The need for stimulation of this sense is satisfied with infant pacifiers, lollipops, gum chewing, and snacking. It is the action of chewing that is satisfying.

Taste and Sweetness

Human beings and animals are pleasure seekers. If an animal is given the choice between a sweet solution or water, it will drink the sweet one and continue to do so until sated. A sweet solution is also pleasant for human beings, as soda manufacturers well know. If you are slim or just mildly overweight, you probably enjoy the concentration of a sweet solution up to a point, at which it will become too sweet for your taste. If you are quite a bit overweight, your body needs a much higher concentration of sweetness, although there is always a point at which a concentrated sweet will become unpleasant. When you feel the need for sweets, you can satiate your sweet "hunger" by providing a sweet concentrated at such a high dosage that it will immediately become unpleasant. For example, chew a saccharin tablet when you crave a sweet. The concentrated sweetness will quickly turn you off. Obviously this should not be done too often—use it only as an emergency measure.

As patients become slimmer, they no longer enjoy concentrated sweet solutions, indicating that their chemistry has been changed. This change helps greatly in keeping weight down unless the patient has excessive insulin, the hormone that regulates the sugar metabolism. Too much insulin produces hypoglycemia (low blood sugar) and increases the desire for sweets. When overweight diabetic animals are injected with insulin and allowed to choose between different sweet solutions, they drink more of the sweetest one. It is not just for pleasure—there is a physiological need in their bodies because their blood-sugar levels are too low. Overweight people have high insulin levels. They usually eat greater quantities of sweets and larger amounts of food but obtain little satisfaction.

Our genetic code signals that sweet tastes are acceptable and bitter tastes are less desirable. I'm going to explain how you can dupe your body to consume fewer sweets. Some tastes clash with each other, so you can play one against the other by chewing a lemon when you want to eat sweets or by having a diet soda if you want to decrease your desire for salty foods.

Water intake has a lot to do with your consumption of sweets. When the water intake of animals is restricted, their sweet intake increases, probably to retain more water. To control your sweet intake, drink lots of water!

Even the temperature of sweet solutions plays a role in the amount of intake. Sweet solutions are more pleasant when very cold or hot; tepid solutions are less desirable. Try drinking soft drinks lukewarm.

> **Drink lots of water and control your sweet tooth.**
>
> **Chew a lemon when you crave sweets.**
>
> **Drink a diet soda to decrease your desire for salty foods.**

Curbing a Sweet Tooth

If you have a sweet tooth, sometimes the urge for sweets means the downfall of your diet as you go on a cookie binge.

To avoid a binge, satisfy the sweet tooth and the need

for chewing with sugarless gum. Choose those containing xylitol—it has no effect on insulin release and is less likely to increase your hunger.

When on an uncontrollable binge, I recommend that you eat the real thing—plain cubes of sugar. As shocking as that might sound, you will be ingesting only 23 calories per cube, and you will eat fewer straight sugar cubes than cookies. Or chew a few sticks of regular gum with sugar. At about 10 calories each, they are a steal! Another way to cool off a binge will be explained on page 37.

Women Are Different

Women's sexual hormones have a lot to do with appetite. There is a dramatic reduction in women's appetite and body weight around the time of ovulation. But many women have noticed that they overeat and gain weight prior to their menstrual period. This cyclical eating is the result of the type and quantity of sexual hormones circulating in the blood during the different stages of a menstrual cycle. A woman should be aware of where she is in her cycle because it is important for the timing of her diet. Start dieting right after a period. There will be three weeks of relatively low appetite, which will help make dieting easier.

TIP FOR WOMEN

Start dieting right after your period. You will have three weeks of relatively low appetite, which will make your dieting easier.

Rational Eating

Your rate of eating also has a lot to do with the frequency of your food intake. The slower you eat your lunch, the later you will eat your dinner. It is okay to have just two meals a day and pass up your morning breakfast, although a light breakfast reduces midmorning snacking. Some patients are content with breakfast and dinner, skipping lunch. You will be in charge of your meal schedule, so observe what your body is telling you about when to eat.

You might know that your stomach distends quickly when you eat fast. When experimental subjects of normal weight eat faster, they eat more. People usually eat fast at the beginning, then slow down and start to enjoy the meal. Pleasure takes over the need for distention. It is important that you become aware of what all my patients know: Make a conscious effort to eat slowly at the beginning of a meal to increase your pleasure and decrease your intake. The best way to accomplish this is to eat some high-fiber foods (listed on page 49) or raw salad as an appetizer. But be aware that high-fiber content does not automatically mean quick satiety.

Several experiments have compared the satiation effect of solid and liquid food. Liquid food provides a degree of satiety comparable to solid food. The catch is that you must drink it slowly! Sip slowly and enjoy your broth, bouillon, or juice 20 minutes prior to your appetizer. Your natural appetite suppressants will be working at top strength by the time you eat your lunch or dinner.

The problem with liquid food is that drinking is too fast and easy. People eat less when their food requires some time and effort to eat.

Do not be too concerned with your stomach noises or pangs. Your stomach muscles are always active and you might have stomach contractions whether you eat a lot, a little, or not at all. When people fast, their smooth gastric muscles contract even without any food to work on. If your stomach makes funny noises due to contractions, don't consider this a call to eat; it is just normal muscle activity.

Eating is less a mental than a chemical reaction. Most of the time there is a chemical force behind your mental needs. This was demonstrated in a recent experiment performed on twenty-five overweight and twenty-three slim women. Tasty, delicious-looking meals were shown to them after several hours of fasting. They were not allowed to eat until some tests were performed. An insulin response stimulated by the sight and smell of the food without eating was four times greater in the overweight women. We know that insulin activates hunger, so this proves the overweights were literally hungrier than the slim. They are chemically programmed to eat!

Body chemistry can be changed. The more information you have about how to remodel it, the more rational the eating process becomes and the greater your chances of controlling your intake. You are well on your way. Keep learning how to play the game.

The Exercise Factor

Exercise should be an important part of every dieter's regimen. It increases the body's metabolic rate, temporarily decreases the appetite, improves circulation of the blood, alleviates stress-related emotions, alters insulin production, and tones your body, which provides motivation to continue dieting. Chapter 5 examines the benefits of exercise and provides simple specific routines that require only 36 minutes a week to maintain fitness.

A Better Way to Relax

Overeating is often a response to stress. Tension influences your eating as well as your choice of food. How you feel often determines what your next food intake will be.

There is an easier way of calming yourself. Tests have shown that anxiety and muscle relaxation are incompatible. If you learn my relaxation technique, discussed in Chapter 6, you can soothe your nerves and maintain control of your eating.

2
What You Should Know Before Starting the Bio-Diet

Composition of Foods

You are indeed what you eat. Foods have specific effects on your body chemistry. You can have the biochemistry of a slim person, absorb few calories, and avoid hunger if you know what to eat and when. Once you have changed your body chemistry, you will be able to stay slim without stringent dieting.

We are going to examine the components of food so you will understand the specific mechanisms of how the body works as well as the scientific roots of the Bio-Diet.

What Happens When You Eat

Food contains six classes of nutrients, all of which are chemicals: carbohydrates, proteins, fats, vitamins, minerals, and water. They interact with your body's chemical enzymes and are broken down before being absorbed and performing their functions.

Carbohydrates are chemical nutrients containing carbon, hydrogen, and oxygen. Simple carbohydrates are glucose, fructose, and galactose. Compound carbohydrates are sucrose, which is found in table sugar, and lactose, which is found in milk. The most complex carbohydrate is starch.

In the intestine, starches and compound carbohydrates are broken down by body enzymes into simple carbohydrates. They are absorbed and deposited in the liver as glycogen, which is changed to glucose and sent to all parts of the body for use as fuel. Insulin delivers glucose to the cells, and any excess glucose is converted into fat.

The feature distinguishing protein from the other chemical nutrients is that it contains nitrogen. Protein is broken down by your body enzymes into amino acids. There are about two dozen amino acids. The body regulates the absorption of amino acids according to their blood level. A low level of the essential amino acid tryptophane will trigger greater absorption of all amino acids.

Amino acids build new body tissue; maintain body structure, enzyme, and hormone production; and regulate the body's water content. Amino acids are sometimes converted into glucose or fat when carbohydrates and fats are unavailable or when there is excessive protein intake.

The main characteristic of fats is that they are insoluble in water. Solid fat comes primarily from animals; oils and liquid fat come from vegetables.

Triglycerides are the basic form of fat we ingest. The churning, kneading, and squirting actions of the stomach turn solid fat triglycerides into a coarse emulsion. Liquid triglycerides reach the intestine even sooner. Bile dissolves triglycerides, and pancreatic enzymes break them into fatty acids. These fatty acids are absorbed by the intestinal cells, then reconverted into triglycerides and delivered to the liver, muscles, and adipose tissue. The liver distributes triglycerides to the body, muscles burn them, and the adipose tissue stores them. Lipoprotein lipase (LPL) is an enzyme that breaks down stored fat when it is needed as fuel.

Vitamins constitute one of the six classes of chemical nutrients. They help in regulating the chemical processes in the body.

Minerals and water are also chemical nutrients. There are fourteen essential minerals, which are all provided by the food of the Bio-Diet.

Water is the most essential nutrient. Although it does not provide any calories for the body, it does provide the medium by which the human body cells perform their metabolic processes. The gastrointestinal system produces as much as 8 or 9 liters of watery fluids per day that are all reabsorbed. These fluids contain the enzymes that break down food as well as some of the substances that regulate the appetite.

When food reaches the stomach and intestine, chemical reactions release hormones that curb the appetite as well as hormones that increase the appetite. Hormones are chemical substances formed in different organs of the body that travel to another part of the body, such as the brain, to produce an action.

Gastric inhibitory peptide (GIP) is an appetite stimulator released by the intake of simple sugars and fats. The main action of GIP is to activate insulin, which in turn decreases blood sugar and increases the appetite.

Abnormally high levels of GIP have been reported in the overweight. It has been noted that after a gastric bypass, a drastic surgical treatment for obesity, GIP has decreased and the ability of food to release insulin has been diminished.

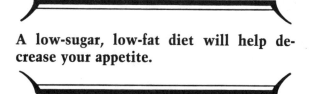

A low-sugar, low-fat diet will help decrease your appetite.

Endorphines, a recently discovered group of hormones, are produced in the stomach and intestine and act like morphine. The name comes from *endo*genous *morphine*. From the intestine, endorphines are transported by the blood to the brain. The type of food that releases endorphines is unknown. Stress will produce an increase in endorphines and changes in the small bowel similar to those produced during fasting.

The injection of purified endorphines produces tranquilization, pain reduction, euphoric changes of mood, and physical dependence. Excessive food and alcoholic intake may produce physical dependence by the release of endorphines. Increased levels of endorphines have been found in the overweight in proportion to body weight.

There are other substances that may also affect appetite. Substance P is a hormone that has been found in the small intestine and the brain. It produces a tranquilization effect similar to endorphine.

Figure 1 on page 21 shows that there are appetite stimulators and appetite depressors. The appetite stimulators are endorphines, GIP, substance P, and insulin. Appetite depressors are tryptophane, serotonin, cholecystokinin (CCK), neurotensin, gastrin, glucagon, and secretin. The quantity of neurotensin released by the intestinal cells is based on the size of the meal. A large volume of food releases more neurotensin, which activates glucagon and slows the emptying of the stomach. Gastrin stimulates gastric juices. It is released by distention and proteins.

Food, therefore, produces chemical reactions and a release of stimulators or depressors of the appetite. The type of food, amount, and order of intake will affect appetite outcome.

Some of the appetite regulators have limited local action and are found only in the gastrointestinal system; others act primarily in the brain.

Natural Appetite Suppressants

When an overweight animal is surgically connected to the arteries and veins of a lean animal of the same species, they share the same blood, nutrients, and chemicals that control their appetites. After several weeks, the overweight animal remains overweight or becomes more obese while the lean animal becomes thinner or dies. Why? Faulty sensors in the brain of the overweight animal don't register the chemicals, and the animal continues to overeat. The lean animal's brain sensors give off signals saying, "We have enough" or "Eat less." The animal stops eating and dies. The overweight animal remains insensitive to the circulating chemicals while the thin one starves because it is too responsive to the chemicals controlling its appetite.

Cholecystokinin is a hormone produced and released in the small intestine after eating and is thought to signal the brain that satiety has been reached. Other regulating hormones are insulin, glucagon, secretin, and thyroid substances.

CCK was discovered years ago but was not known to have any role in appetite control. This hormone was known to have the property of emptying the gallbladder to help digest food. It was found recently that when food enters the small intestine, the level of CCK increases to its highest point, and the subject feels satiated. From that result, it was concluded that CCK signals satiation. This was recently confirmed by injecting purified CCK into sixteen hungry overweight persons who were watching the preparation of a delicious meal. The people rated their degree of hunger, and the CCK was shown to have markedly decreased their appetite.

CCK appears to act directly on the brain, acting as a messenger saying, "Stop eating. I'm full." Experiments at Mount Sinai School of Medicine in New York found that the brains of overweight mice contained less CCK than the brains of slim mice.

Proteins and fats are the specific food components that increase CCK. When the proteins and fats are in solid form, it takes longer to increase the level of CCK. The maximum level of CCK is obtained when you drink a solution of proteins or fatty fluids such as soups, broths, and acidic juices. This new knowledge about CCK is a major factor in my dieting program. The trick is to curb your appetite without adding too many calories. Increase your CCK levels by drinking proteins or fatty fluids before beginning a meal. You will feel satisfied soon after starting your actual meal and will decrease the amount of food you eat.

Stomach acid juices also increase CCK. Because tea and coffee are stomach acid stimulators, you can use them to limit food intake. Robert S., one of my patients who lost 40 pounds, has become an expert in this technique. He drinks a cup of coffee black or with a little skim milk before meals. At a restaurant, he has a cup of coffee before ordering. Then he eats with gusto, enjoying his meals to the maximum, but without overeating.

Humans eat more when confronted with physical and emotional pain. CCK can control your psychological eating.

Some doctors believe that a natural protein component called tryptophane will help produce satiety if taken before eating solid food. It is available in tablets at health stores and pharmacies. Tryptophane has a triple effect: It seems to increase CCK, curb the sweet tooth, and release the brain chemical serotonin. Serotonin also affects your eating behavior by reducing the appetite and prolonging the amount of time between meals. Serotonin increases after any aerobic exercise.

Fresh grapefruit, lemon, or lime juice is also effective. Acidic juices release secretin from the upper intestine. Secretin increases pancreatic juices and enzymes that act upon ingested fats, which in turn activate CCK. Drink the juice slowly before your main course, drink a large glass of water, and enjoy your food. The water speeds up the passage of acid from the stomach into the intestine, where CCK is released. Drink fluids at the beginning of a meal so you will start eating with a semifull stomach. Drinking water, tea, or diet sodas between meals also helps keep the CCK at a good level because gastric acid juices are flushed into the bowel and produce CCK.

TWO IMPORTANT HORMONES

Insulin and glucagon are two other important hormones involved with appetite control. They are both produced in the pancreas but have opposite effects on the body's blood-sugar level. When insulin goes up, blood sugar goes down, which triggers the release of glucagon. When glucagon goes up, it raises a low blood-sugar level, thereby calming hunger. Glucagon also helps break down fat and increases the level of ketones, which curb the appetite. Ketones are by-products of fat breakdown.

Overweight people frequently have a low level of glucagon, so it is important to increase it by natural methods. Fasting, eating proteins, and exercising increase the glucagon levels in your body. Birth-control pills or a large sugar intake decrease them.

> **Increase your CCK levels before beginning a meal. Twenty minutes before you eat, have a small cup of chicken broth with fat, tomato juice, 2 capsules of safflower oil, or a glass of fresh grapefruit, lemon, or lime juice. A cup of tea or coffee with or without skim milk will activate CCK too. The sooner your natural appetite suppressants are released, the better. And don't forget to drink plenty of fluids before each meal. Have one tablet of tryptophane between meals.**

After eating sweets, the insulin level increases in the blood, and CCK is *not* released. Then the insulin level drops sharply. When your insulin level drops quickly, your appetite increases. One of the most important points in dieting is to choose foods carefully to avoid this dramatic rise and fall of insulin level. For instance, if you have to choose between eating rice, potatoes, or bread, you will probably eat the one you think is least damaging, presumably potatoes. You are close, but not exactly correct. Rice increases the insulin level gradually and decreases it gently. Bread produces a sharp increase and a plunging drop of the insulin level. The effect of eating potatoes falls somewhere in the middle. Eating bread will make you feel hungry sooner because your insulin level drops quickly. Nutritionally, brown rice is even better than white rice because it still contains the fiber, which is removed during processing.

> **Carefully choose foods to avoid a dramatic rise and fall of insulin level. If you have the choice of eating rice, potatoes, or bread, pick rice. It gradually increases your insulin level, which then gently decreases.**

Using Your Body Chemistry to Your Advantage

The most active part of thyroid hormones is called T-3. Its most important function is burning calories by working upon an enzyme called ATPase, which consumes energy.

In 1980, a widely published medical report found that overweights burn fewer calories than slim people because of faulty ATPase activity. Whether you have faulty ATPase function or normal, a prescription for T-3 is not the solution because it will increase your appetite. The excessive use of thyroid pills might result in exactly what you don't want—overeating—while the benefits might be nil. Aerobic exercise activates ATPase without increasing your appetite. Low salt and high potassium intake—fruits and vegetables are good sources of potassium—also activate ATPase.

The Bio-Diet and Your Appetite

My diet, relaxation, and exercise program will affect the interplay of substances in the following manner:
1. Increase appetite suppressors
   a. The early intake of liquid oils or acid juices releases CCK and secretin.
   b. Soluble fiber and vegetables, which increase the bulk in the stomach and intestines, release neurotensin and gastrin.
   c. Proteins with low fat release gastrin, provide tryptophane, and increase glucagon.
   d. Serotonin is increased by aerobic exercise and tryptophane.
2. Avoid appetite stimulators
   a. Reduction of intake of simple sugars and solid fats decreases the likelihood of large GIP and insulin release.
   b. Stress release of endorphines is neutralized by the use of the relaxation reflex.

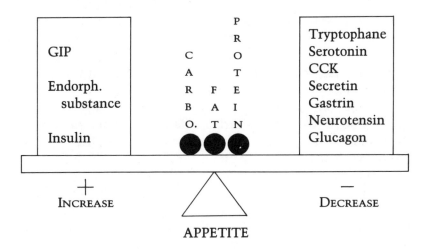

How and what you eat increases or decreases your appetite.

Because carbohydrates provide the major portion of calories in the average diet, it is an appropriate beginning to the discussion of food components.

Carbohydrates

Lactose from milk and sucrose in table sugar are two sugars that are rapidly absorbed and transformed into glucose (blood sugar). The rapid absorption of these simple sugars quickly increases your circulating glucose, which triggers the release of insulin to bring it back down. Insulin increases fat deposits and reduces glucose in your blood, which then increases hunger. Obviously, sudden insulin release is most unwanted.

HOW GOOD IS THE SUGAR IN FRUITS?

Fructose is a simple sugar that is locked into fruits and vegetables. It has a lower rate of absorption than lactose or sucrose. Fructose is absorbed according to its concentration in the intestine—the larger the amount ingested, the higher the absorption. Fructose usually does not trigger a rapid release of insulin in your blood, except in large amounts or when mixed with other sugars. Fruits and vegetables are less troublesome than table sugar, but an excessive intake will disturb a balanced biochemistry. One apple is fine but three are almost as bad as a slice of cake. Too much fructose will make you gain weight almost as easily as too much refined sugar. If you eat an apple, your insulin level rises a little and goes down slowly. If you have applesauce, a higher level of insulin is produced. But when you drink a glass of apple juice, your insulin level jumps up as rapidly as if you had consumed a soda. A high-fructose diet can produce chronic diarrhea, colic, and gas.

HOW FATTENING IS MILK?

Milk is a two-edged sword: It increases insulin rapidly, but its proteins and calcium help decrease your appetite. My conclusion is that drinking milk in small amounts (2 to 4 ounces) is beneficial, especially when added to coffee or tea. Skim milk has less fat than regular milk but contains the same amount of sugar. Remember the story of the Turkish sultan who loved obese slaves and kept his beauties overweight by frequently feeding them large amounts of milk!

LOW-CARBOHYDRATE DIETS CAN TURN OFF YOUR THYROID!

Sugar has 4 calories per gram, alcohol has 7, and fat 9. Because of its lower caloric content, sugar per se is less fattening than alcohol or cream cheese. Cutting down the carbohydrate content of the diet for a long time decreases thyroid activity, which lowers metabolism. Energy level is lower too. These unwanted effects are more marked when the diet is very low in calories.

My diet will manipulate carbohydrate consumption to your best advantage while keeping your thyroid working well. You will be eating starches and other complex carbohydrates but avoiding refined simple sugars.

Starches are the most complex carbohydrates. Flour is the best-known processed starch. The more processed a starch is, the more quickly it is absorbed and the greater insulin reaction it produces. For example, if you eat an ear of corn, your insulin level will increase quickly, but not as quickly as it would if you have gravy made with processed corn starch.

The digestibility or level of absorption of a purified starch is 100 percent, whereas the same starch in its natural state is absorbed only 93 percent. By eating fiber in conjunction with a processed starch, such as broccoli with noodles, you can decrease carbohydrate absorption markedly. When carbohydrate absorption is delayed, it decreases food consumption, which in turn affects body weight and body fat.

> **Always eat fibers in conjunction with starches to decrease carbohydrate absorption.**

Glycogen is the form in which carbohydrates are stored in the muscles and liver. When there is too much glycogen stored in the body, subsequent absorbed sugars are turned into fat. Glycogen and fat can be used for energy. When you undertake moderate exercise, you quickly use up the glycogen stored in muscles and the liver and begin to burn up fat. To stay slim, you must eat moderate amounts of carbohydrates and exercise regularly to use up some of the stored glycogen.

VISIBLE AND INVISIBLE SUGARS

You are probably eating excessive sugar and purified starches without even being aware of it. Most processed foods contain surprising quantities of devalued and unnecessary carbohydrates. They are disguised as modified food starch, modified corn starch, corn syrup, and dextrin.

Processed foods are not allowed on my diet, which emphasizes good, simple, and natural foods. This doesn't mean that the Bio-Diet is tasteless or boring. We know that an appealing, tasty diet has more chance of success than a bland one. The sight, smell, and taste of food produce a physiological effect on the secretion of digestive juices. Early release of digestive juices by appealing food produces the quickest satiation, thereby signaling an early end to your eating. I believe you should enjoy yourself as much as possible while dieting. You will probably appreciate food *more* when you can control its effects on your body chemistry. Learn to use new flavors and spices—garlic, red and black pepper, rosemary, and curry powder can add another dimension to food preparation and enjoyment.

Soluble Fiber

The digestive juices break down plant food for the absorption of nutrients. However, there are food constituents such as cellulose that are resistant to digestion. They are the skeletal remains of vegetable cells and are known as roughage. Vegetables and fruits have another fiber that is digested by the stomach juices and becomes a gel—it is called soluble fiber. Soluble fiber and roughage act differently in the digestive system. Roughage speeds up transit through the intestines; soluble-fiber gel slows it down. By eating foods containing proportionally more soluble fiber than roughage, you can decrease the intake and absorption of calories. The right mix of soluble fiber and roughage does three things: (1) It occupies more space in the stomach and intestines, allowing less room for other food because part of the fiber is not absorbed. (2) It requires more chewing, slowing down food consumption and increasing saliva and gastric secretions, which swell the fiber, distend the stomach, and produce a full feeling. (3) The soluble-fiber gel reduces absorption in the intestine and slows down the transit of the food. This has been demonstrated by providing soluble fiber to patients ingesting fats, proteins, and carbohydrates. When soluble fiber was included in the diet, stool elimination of all these caloric substances was highest. Soluble fiber lowers fat absorption from 85 to 95 percent down to 54 to 62 percent. Fat has 9 calories and fiber close to 0, so you will save caloric absorption by having soluble fiber before fat intake.

Eating soluble fiber decreases sugar absorption. There

is not a dramatic release of insulin, which avoids a drop in blood glucose and an increase in hunger or fat deposits. Protein absorption also decreases.

HOW SOLUBLE FIBER WORKS

A current diet proclaims the following benefits from eating large quantities of roughage: decreased likelihood of colon cancer, bowel diverticular disease (small herniations), nervous bowel, appendicitis, hemorrhoids, and varicose veins. Soluble fiber, which is favored on my diet, is of benefit for gallstones, diabetes mellitus, and arteriosclerotic heart disease.

Soluble fiber has no known drawbacks. Unfortunately, there are some problems with large quantities of roughage—it can produce an excessive amount of gas and diarrhea as well as decrease the absorption of important vitamins and minerals such as B_{12}, calcium, iron, and zinc.

> **Eat slowly at the beginning of a meal. Have high-fiber vegetables or raw salad for an appetizer.**

Soluble fiber blocks the absorption of fat and sugar while leaving vitamin metabolism unaltered. This discovery was made when doctors were studying the effects of soluble fiber on heart disease. The test group ate well but absorbed food poorly and lost weight. It was concluded that the weight loss was due to less efficient digestion. Soluble-fiber gel coating the stomach and intestines had blocked caloric absorption.

The Bio-Diet provides sufficient soluble fiber to achieve the lowest level of caloric absorption. There are moderate amounts of roughage balanced with other nutrients to obtain the benefits of fiber without the side effects.

> Eat foods with a higher soluble-fiber content to decrease the absorption of calories. Add pulverized rind of citrus fruits to juice for extra pectin, the key soluble fiber.

THE KEY SOLUBLE FIBER: PECTIN

Pectin is a soluble fiber found in fruits and some vegetables. Pectin has very important properties. It decreases the absorption of cholesterol, lowering blood cholesterol levels. It decreases the insulin-releasing action of carbohydrates, thus helping in appetite control. When volunteers ate most of their carbohydrates as refined sugars, they complained of hunger, but when they ate the same quantity of carbohydrates in vegetables and fruits containing pectin, they felt stuffed.

Pectin and some roughage have the capacity of holding water in the intestines. The more water retained from the foods you eat, the more volume in your bowels, which distends the gastrointestinal system and gives satisfaction. Large food volume activates two hormones: gastrin in the stomach and neurotensin in the intestine. They release glucagon and gastric juices and slow stomach emptying time.

Pectin has the highest water-holding capacity. Bran has high water-holding capacity and leaves the intestines without being digested, but it can produce diarrhea. Carrots also have good water-holding capacity. Almost 600 grams of potatoes are needed to achieve the same water-holding capacity as 100 grams of raw carrots.

But the most important property of pectin is that it

saves calories because it decreases the absorption of fat. The amount of fat lost in the stools when ingesting pectin ranges from 2 to 43 percent. Failing to absorb 40 percent of your fat intake means a substantial savings in calories. If you don't absorb the fat, you don't absorb the calories. Pectin is the key.

The rind of citrus fruits is 30 percent pectin. A blender can help you get more pectin—just throw part of the rind of the grapefruit into the blender when you make fresh juice. Drink it before your meals and you will save calories!

Pectin is soluble in hot water, so vegetables high in this soluble fiber are depleted and worthless after being boiled. I provide a list of vegetables high in soluble fiber and pectin with good water-holding capacity on page 49. Do not boil them!

The Pattern of Intake

The most important part of my diet is the timed intake of soluble fiber, pectin, and other nutrients. I have found that soluble fiber and pectin must be taken after the initial liquid intake (see page 46) and right before eating any carbohydrates and proteins. For instance, at dinnertime, after a cup of broth, enjoy a salad with vegetables from the soluble-fiber list. You can supplement this with 2 tablets of apple pectin. The second dish of the meal can be cooked vegetables. The meal ends with a small quantity of proteins and carbohydrates such as fish or noodles.

This pattern of intake encourages lots of chewing, an early release of digestive juices, maximum feelings of satisfaction, minimum caloric intake, and low food absorption.

The Good and Bad of Protein

Even though protein intake is listed toward the end of the meal, protein is probably the most important substance in your food intake. It is eaten at the end of the meal because it prolongs the interval between meals through its action on the hormones that affect the appetite. Protein releases gastrin, a hormone that stimulates stomach acid secretion, glucagon, CCK, and others that produce a feeling of satiety. When protein is broken down by digestive juices, it becomes amino acids, which is what your body absorbs and uses to build new body tissue and maintain body structure. Because proteins are lost from the body in urine and feces, they must be readily replenished.

Eggs, milk, and meats are complete proteins with all the essential amino acids necessary for good nutrition. Eggs provide the best-quality protein but are considered too high in cholesterol to consume often. Beans, peas, and nuts, for instance, are incomplete proteins. Mother's milk has the perfect mixture of amino acids. If eggs are considered 100 percent ideal protein, cow's milk, meat, and fish are only 75 percent as good, rice 60 percent, beans and peas .4 percent, and gelatin 0.

When you eat more protein than your body needs, the amino acids are removed by the liver and converted to urea, which is excreted by the kidneys. An excess of urea increases urine output, which expels essential minerals and can lead to dehydration. On a high-protein diet, you might show a large initial weight loss that is not due to fat breakdown but to excessive urine output. When the kidney function is reduced because of illness or age, high-protein intake can lead to uremia, increased toxins in the blood. Any extra protein will be utilized by the body as calories instead of being subtracted from your fat deposits.

What is the ideal amount of protein? The answer is still in question. Nutritionists in the United States, Japan, and West Germany do not yet agree on a figure. This diet meets the U.S. requirements.

The availability of amino acids in a protein source like meat are decreased by broiling. In the browned outer part of roast meat, the amino acids link in forms that cannot be absorbed. So the browning reaction adds flavor to your meat and reduces the amount of amino acids to be absorbed. Toasting also reduces the absorption of bread carbohydrates. Toast a thin slice of bread at the darkest setting. Yes, your grandmother was right!

Proteins should be taken with as little fat as possible because fats and proteins together can *increase* your weight. Peanuts are an excellent source of protein, iron, and vitamins, but they contain too much fat. Most nuts are not allowed on my diet. I have allowed 1 tablespoon (15 grams) of peanut butter for breakfast. This equals the caloric value of one hard-cooked egg. It will keep you satiated until lunch, thus avoiding a midmorning snack.

Choose the leanest cuts of meat from the list on page 51. *Most fish and poultry are lower in fat and should be used instead of meat whenever possible.* My patients have better results when they eat less red meat and more fish and poultry.

> **Broiling meats reduces the amino acids that can be absorbed by the body. When you begin eating bread after attaining your weight goal, toast it to decrease the absorption of carbohydrates.**

Fat Intake and Fat Deposits

Adipose tissues (fatty deposits) are the caloric reservoir of the body. Adipose tissue is depleted by eating fewer calories than your body requires, consuming calories and exercising, or both. But you might have some biochemical resistance or physiological blocks to weight loss.

First, you can have an excessive amount of circulating insulin, which quickly transforms the carbohydrate intake into fat. Second, the enzymes that break down the fat of your adipose tissues might be malfunctioning. Third, the fat material in your adipose tissue can be hard to break down, especially if you eat a lot of meat, cheese, and junk food. Fourth, your muscles might not be consuming enough calories due to atrophy. Finally, your metabolism could be slower than normal because of a hormonal dysfunction or older age.

You might have few or all of these problems coupled with the psychological hang-up of being overweight. You might have tried every possible new diet. No wonder you are so skeptical about losing fat. My program will remove all of the stumbling blocks except, of course, your age.

EXCESSIVE INSULIN

It is likely that you have a high level of this hormone due to your past eating habits, and you must learn how to get it down to normal levels. In fact, your body is probably resistant to insulin and that is why your pancreas makes more of it to balance your system. Don't worry. Insulin can be decreased simply by exercise and diet. The closer to normal your insulin level becomes, the more fat you are going to lose.

ENZYME MALFUNCTION

Lipoprotein lipase (LPL), an enzyme that breaks down the fat tissue, is less active in overweight people. It somehow facilitates losing weight. Caffeine might be a factor in the malfunction of LPL, so watch your coffee consumption. Exercise and fasting improve the LPL function.

FAT BREAKDOWN

The types of fat you eat have a lot to do with the type of fat deposited in your adipose tissue. There are basically two types of fats you should be aware of—unsaturated and saturated. Unsaturated fats are found in safflower, sunflower, corn, and walnut oils and are helpful in decreasing cholesterol in your blood. Unsaturated oils given to rats produced fewer fat cells than saturated fats. When deposited in the adipose tissue, they can be easily broken down.

Saturated fats are found in meats, milk products such as butter and cheese, and vegetable shortening. When absorbed, they increase the cholesterol level and are harder to lose when converted to adipose tissue. Junk food is packed with saturated fats. Buy oils high in polyunsaturated fats and do not be afraid to use it to fry your fish—it's perfectly all right to fry protein food twice a week, though broiling is better.

EAT A LITTLE FAT TO LOSE FAT!

Fat intake is absolutely necessary to avoid malnutrition because certain vitamins require fat to be absorbed. If you follow a fat-free diet, 30 percent of your ingested carbohydrates will be converted into fat and deposited in your adipose tissue. On the other hand, small amounts of fat in the diet curb the appetite and strongly inhibit the adiposity buildup produced by sugar intake. Large amounts of fat have the opposite effect—they increase weight and hunger. There seems to be no limit to the ability of the body to store fat.

Liquid unsaturated fats such as safflower and corn oil and fats from chicken or beef broth release the appetite-control hormones faster than their solid counterparts. Avoid solid forms of fat by trimming meats and poultry skin, which provide calories without curbing your appetite. All cold cuts, processed meats, and junk foods contain excessive fat. Turkey rolls, corned beef, frankfurters, pizza, and potato chips are examples of foods that will increase your appetite by raising your insulin level. By consuming liquid oils such as those found in soups and by staying away from solid animal fats, you will decrease your cholesterol intake and curb your hunger. If you dislike soups and broths, take 2 capsules of safflower oil about 20 minutes before meals.

MUSCLES AND CALORIES

When your muscles work, they consume up to 75 percent of your caloric intake. You must stimulate the system that burns your food transgressions! Aerobic exercise activates the enzyme ATPase, which uses up calories in every cell of the body. Exercise is especially important to stay slim once you have your weight down.

METABOLIC SLOWDOWN

You might have been told, or you are hoping, that your metabolic rate is at fault. There is considerable controversy as to whether the overweight person has a decreased metabolic rate. Studies have found that an overweight person can be in good health and active while using half the calories of a slim person. Also, when sleeping, overweights burn fewer calories than their slim counterparts. It seems unfair.

Weather is a factor in metabolism. A cold environment increases the metabolic rate of slim persons while not increasing that of overweight people because the overweights are protected by their fat. On the other hand, after losing weight, the formerly fat are more affected by the cold due to an inability to raise their body temperatures.

Overweight people often have huge weight gain when they increase their sugar intake. What is even worse, when overweight people go onto a very-low-calorie diet for more than eight days, their metabolic rate goes down another 10 to 15 percent. Slow weight loss is the result, and many dieters give up. To counteract the slower metabolism, a dieter must cut down intake even more or exercise harder.

This often proves to be overwhelming, and the majority quit and go back to overeating. But what if your metabolic blood tests are normal and the "sluggish" thyroid passes with flying colors? The fact is that fewer than 5 percent of the overweight patients referred to endocrine clinics have a significantly low metabolism. The deficiency might be in your body cells and not in your thyroid gland. The most recently discovered factor is the enzyme called ATPase.

All the cells of your body have the ATPase enzyme (page 20), which pumps sodium from inside the cell into the surrounding fluids and maintains potassium levels inside the cells. This enzyme consumes lots of calories—from 20 to 50 percent of the body's total expenditure. One method of measuring how well this enzyme functions and how many calories are being burned is to find out how much sodium is left in the cell. An excessive amount of sodium indicates a deficient "pumping" system that uses few calories. Overweights were found to have excessive sodium in their cells and lower ATPase activity. This could be the reason why even when you eat very little you don't lose, or when you eat an average amount you gain. Diuretics (water pills) do not help to decrease your cellular sodium. Aerobic exercise does it!

YOUR METABOLIC RATE CAN CHANGE

All metabolic systems eventually slow down with age. Women over forty find it more difficult to lose weight than men because the female metabolism is 10 percent lower. But don't lose hope. What we know today might not be true tomorrow. For instance, it was once thought that people who had been overweight since childhood had more fat cells than those who became overweight as adults. Though this is often true, the reverse is also possible—fat cells can decrease in number in adulthood.

Exercise is an excellent way to improve your metabolic rate without drugs. Exercise releases adrenaline, which activates ATPase, triggering the pumping action that burns calories. Cigarettes and caffeine also increase your metabolic rate. Caffeine has a dual action: It increases the metabolic rate, but it can block enzymes that break down fat. I feel that a moderate amount of caffeine is not harmful, and it is allowed on my diet. Cigarette smoking is a dangerous way to improve your metabolism, and it is not recommended.

> **Exercise releases adrenaline, which activates ATPase.**

It is still debatable whether thyroid medication helps, and more research is needed on this subject.

How to Prolong Morning Satiation

Fasting lowers the insulin level, while glucagon (the hormone opposite in effect to insulin) remains high. The change in concentration of these hormones releases fat from the adipose tissue. If there are no carbohydrates available, the released fat produces ketones. After a twelve-hour overnight fast, the ketone level is three times greater than the after-eating level. This chemical reaction keeps you free of morning hunger.

With the first intake of carbohydrates such as a sandwich, a bagel, or a pizza, the glucagon and ketones drop, insulin increases, and you get hungry. The standard pattern is to alternate periods of hunger and eating all through the day.

The Bio-Diet is constructed to prolong morning satiation as long as possible. The best way to do this is to ingest a small amount of protein as your first solid food of the day. It will not decrease glucagon or ketones, and your morning satiation will be prolonged. Starches are consumed later on and simple sugars are avoided. One small piece of fruit before eating protein is allowed.

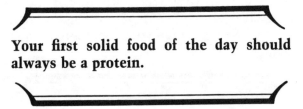

Your first solid food of the day should always be a protein.

Water Intake and Water Retention

The following cases illustrate how water retention is caused by sugar or starch intake: An overweight man who had been losing weight successfully on a prescribed diet was given a large sugar intake for two days. The man suddenly gained 18 pounds, which required three weeks to lose. The weight gain was water.

Hormones and other factors can also cause water retention. Many women complain of their tendency to retain water. This problem is common in 5 to 10 percent of all women, and as many as 30 percent may be mildly affected. The retention is usually triggered by the menses, stress, or hot weather.

Before every period, Mrs. S. gained an average of 3 to 5 pounds. Her hands and legs swelled, and she suffered headaches, anxiety, depression, and epigastric bloating. Swelling and other symptoms were decreased by rest and a low-salt diet.

Excessive water retention can be controlled by intelligent dieting. You can eat a moderate amount of starches intermittently before and during ovulation, but avoid carbohydrates before the onset of menstruation. Urination will increase and swelling will be relieved by restricting salt, lying down during day rest periods, and wearing support panty hose.

> **TIP FOR WOMEN**
>
> To reduce water retention before your period, avoid carbohydrates, restrict salt intake, rest, and wear support panty hose.

Eating Control Through "Natural Food Supplements"

Safflower oil capsules, pectin tablets, and tryptophane tablets may be used in conjunction with the Bio-Diet. They can help but are *not* absolutely necessary to lose weight. Use the lowest dose that works for you. Discontinue food supplements as soon as your appetite is under control.

I have already explained how to increase CCK, one of the hormones that curbs the appetite, by taking safflower oil and tryptophane, and that pectin forms a gel that decreases caloric absorption. They are sold over the counter at pharmacies and health stores. To curb your appetite, take 1 or 2 capsules of safflower oil with grapefruit, lemon, lime, tomato, or vegetable juice approximately 20 minutes before meals. Supplement the amount of soluble fiber in your vegetables with 2 tablets of apple pectin before the main dish to decrease the absorption of fat intake. Take 1 tablet (500 mg) of tryptophane between meals to curb a sweet tooth and to increase satiation. Follow the diet and enjoy the results!

This knowledge can be used to control a binge too! As soon as you feel like starting to nibble and realize that you might be unable to stop, try to relax (see page 129), and swallow 2 capsules of safflower oil, 1 tablet of tryptophane, and 2 tablets of apple pectin. Drink lots of the allowed fluids (page 47) and start a strenuous activity. It works—you will lost interest in food!

Some people have incorporated this "emergency" treatment into their daily eating routine to control their appetites while eating junk food. I do not approve of this. While it is possible not to follow a diet and still lose weight, you must understand that this is not a desirable approach to weight control. Abuse of this external appetite control through natural food supplements induces excessive consumption of food.

> **Curb your appetite by taking 1 or 2 capsules of safflower oil with grapefruit, lemon, lime, tomato, or vegetable juice approximately 20 minutes before meals.**

Those who are opposed to taking any kind of pills should have a cup of soup or broth 20 minutes before a meal and then drink a glass of grapefruit, lemon, lime, tomato, or vegetable juice with pulverized rind (see page 47) at mealtime. Orange and other fruit juices are not allowed because of their high sugar content and low acidity.

It's Time to Diet

Now you know the scientific basis of the Bio-Diet. And you are ready to begin. Remember, you can reduce your appetite and lose weight by following this Bio-Diet plan. But there are three parts to controlling your body chemistry and eventually changing it:

1. Begin the Bio-Diet—Chapter 3.
2. Start the special exercise program using interval exercises—Chapter 4.
3. Control stress using the relaxation reflex—Chapter 5.

3
The Bio-Diet

There are hundreds of diets to help you lose weight. Some are good and some are bad, but many are dangerous. Some reducing diets are based on medical grounds, others are fads, and some try to change your behavior. My diet was developed after years of analyzing and applying the latest research in physiology, chemistry, and psychology, in combination with my personal experience as a bariatric physician, specializing in treatment of the overweight.

We all know that a low-calorie regimen (lower than the amount usually consumed) is all that is needed to lose weight. But there are two other important considerations: First, there is the need to stay on a low-calorie diet long enough to get results, and second, the need to avoid hunger. Most diets fail for one or the other of these factors. They either bore you or cause you to feel starved. These conditions are not conducive to long-term dieting.

My diet offers between 800 and 1,000 calories a day. You can choose among different meats, vegetables, and starches, so you will not be bored. Also, my diet increases the natural body chemicals that control your appetite; therefore, you will not feel hungry.

One dieting problem is the short motivation span. After the first week on a diet, cheating starts, guilt feelings follow, and we quit to stop the self-punishment. On the Bio-Diet, after one week of hard work, you will get a break week, which allows starches and fruits. Good, satisfying, tasty food is never more than one week away, so you will be motivated to avoid cheating during the work week. On the break week, you can legally cheat. When the week is over, you will be ready to begin working seriously again on another work week.

Diets that require the preparation of special meals can be followed at home, but they become a chore for the average working person. On the Bio-Diet you can eat at cafeterias, diners, or restaurants because the diet consists of commonly available foods. There are no unreasonable restrictions. I have provided lists of proteins (page 51), vegetables (pages 49–50), fruits (page 53), and fluids (page 47). Select any foods on those lists for more flexibility in dieting—it permits you to work with the foods that are available.

The Bio-Diet: One Week Work, One Week Fun

There are two weekly plans on the Bio-Diet. The first is a "work week"; the second is a "break week." You can speed up your fat loss by following only the frugal work-week diet, or can slow it down by adding a break week.

During a work week, your food is limited to a low-calorie plan of vegetables, proteins, and fluids. During a break week, you are allowed all that you have on a work week plus selected fruits, starches (pasta, rice, or potatoes), and simple sugars (candied orange or grapefruit peel).

You should start the Bio-Diet with a work week. At the end of the first work week you can follow with another work week to lose weight more quickly or take a breather with a break week. *If your doctor allows, stay on the work-week plan as long as you want.* When you want a change, start a break week. At the end of every break week, you must return to a work-week diet. Do not take two break weeks in a row. You can alternate between work weeks and break weeks, but remember not to have two break weeks in a row.

The Bio-Diet provides for three meals a day, but any meal can be skipped if that is your usual pattern of eating. *You must have at least two meals a day.* Do not have seconds of anything but vegetables.

THE FIRST FEW MINUTES OF A MEAL ARE VERY IMPORTANT

The total amount of food you eat is the direct result of what you do in the first few minutes of a meal. Use those first minutes wisely to obtain the following:

1. A flushing of acidic juices into the intestines to release the hormones that control the appetite. This is done by drinking acidic fluids—grapefruit, lemon, lime, tomato, vegetable juices—before the meal.
2. Early CCK release, which occurs after drinking broth, bouillon, consommé.
3. A low-caloric intake during the first part of the meal, which results from having vegetables and fruits that are low in calories and high in soluble fiber as the first dish.
4. Decreased absorption of foods. Your first dish of fruits and vegetables will provide a large amount of soluble fiber, which will decrease the absorption of fats and carbohydrates in your second dish. Vegetables and fruits containing soluble fiber are listed on pages 49, 50, and 53. The vegetables at the top of the list are preferred.
5. Increased stomach distention and release of appetite-suppressing hormones, which are induced by eating water-retaining fruits or vegetables (pages 49 and 53).

Bio-Diet Work Weeks

BREAKFAST

- Unlimited amounts of low-caloric fluids (page 47). Skim milk can be added to coffee or tea.
- One small fruit or a small glass of fruit juice from lists on pages 47 and 53.

- A 1-ounce portion of protein (page 52). For example, 1 slice (or 1 ounce) of cheese, 1 tablespoon of peanut butter, 2 tablespoons of plain yogurt or cottage cheese, or 1 egg any style.
- Take 1 capsule of multiple vitamins with minerals.

LUNCH

- Drink 1 cup of a caloric fluid (page 47) 20 minutes before lunch or take 1 or 2 capsules of safflower oil.
- Begin with lots of starter vegetables (page 49). Take 2 tablets of pectin.
- Follow with a filler vegetable (page 50) if still hungry. Eat enough to feel satiated. Filler vegetables and proteins are optional at lunch. If you feel the need to snack before dinner, you probably need proteins at lunch. You can eat double the amount of protein at dinner if you pass it up at lunch.

  You should not eat vegetables and proteins at the same time. Starters and fillers are eaten first, then followed with the protein. This rule also applies at dinner.
- End the meal with 4 ounces of any protein (page 51).

SNACKS

- Diet gelatin and any of the listed caloric and noncaloric fluids are okay. Do not eat any solid food.
- Take 1 tablet of tryptophane.

DINNER

- Drink 8 ounces of a caloric fluid (page 47) or take 1 or 2 capsules of safflower oil 20 minutes before the meal.
- Begin with lots of a starter vegetable (page 49). Take 2 tablets of apple pectin.

- Follow with a filler vegetable (page 50) until satiated.
- 4 ounces of protein (page 51) end the meal.

Bio-Diet Break Weeks

BREAKFAST

- Same as work week (see page 43).

LUNCH

- Drink 1 cup of a caloric fluid (page 47) 20 minutes before lunch or take 1 or 2 capsules of safflower oil. Soups are allowed when one-third solid and two-thirds water.
- Begin with lots of starter vegetables (page 49). One serving of allowed fruits (page 53) can be substituted as first dish. Take 2 tablets of apple pectin.
- Follow with a filler vegetable (page 50) if still hungry. This is optional.
- Then have a starch (rice, potatoes, noodles, or macaronis) with allowed sauces (page 52). This is optional.
- End the meal with 4 ounces of a protein (page 51). If you have a starch, fish, poultry, and shellfish are allowed. *Do not eat red meat with starches.* Proteins are optional at lunch.

SNACKS

- Diet gelatin and any of the caloric and noncaloric fluids are okay. Do not eat any solid food.
- Take 1 tablet of tryptophane.

DINNER

- Drink 1 cup of a caloric fluid or 1 glass of a noncaloric fluid (page 47) and take 1 or 2 capsules of safflower oil 20 minutes before dinner.
- Begin with lots of a starter vegetable (page 49). Take 2 tablets of pectin. Allowed fruits (page 53) can be substituted as first dish.
- Follow with a filler vegetable if still hungry (page 50).
- Have 1 serving of starch (rice, potatoes, noodles, or macaronis) as a side or main dish with allowed sauces. This is optional.
- Then have 4 ounces of protein (page 51) or 8 ounces if you did not have protein at lunch. If you have a starch, fish, poultry, and shellfish are allowed. Do not eat red meat with starches.
- Candied orange or grapefruit peels are allowed when you desire a sweet after dinner.

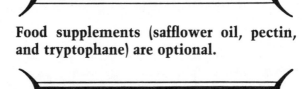

Food supplements (safflower oil, pectin, and tryptophane) are optional.

Diet Components

FLUIDS

You can drink unlimited amounts of water, diet soda, and other noncaloric fluids at any time. Caloric fluids must be ingested before a meal and can be used as a snack in limited amounts. The lists of noncaloric and caloric fluids follow.

One cup of soup without crackers is allowed on break weeks. The solids in the soup should be less than one-third the total volume. Cream soups are allowed only if diluted

50 percent with water. Green pea, split pea, and bean and ham soups are not allowed due to their high caloric content.

Take 1 or 2 capsules of safflower oil with vegetable juices to increase their satiation value.

Allowed Fluids

A. Low-Caloric (Unlimited amounts are allowed at any time before, during, or after a meal.)

> Water
> Tea (no sugar or honey can be added)
> Coffee and decaffeinated coffee (no sugar or honey can be added)
> Mineral water
> Seltzer
> Diet sodas

B. Caloric (Drink before a meal or as a snack. Limited to 1 cup per meal or snack.)

> Beef broth
> Bouillon
> Consommé
> Chicken consommé
> Consommé madrilene
> Clam juice
> Grapefruit juice
> Vegetable juice
> Mixed vegetable juice (V-8, etc.)
> Lemon or lime juice and water
> Tomato juice
> Dietetic or low-calorie gelatin

Safflower oil Take 1–2 capsules or 2–4 pellets before meals with glass of water or juices listed above or add a few drops of safflower oil to the caloric fluids for quick satiation.

VEGETABLES

Most vegetables are allowed on the Bio-Diet. Those excluded are too high in calories and carbohydrates or too low in soluble fiber and water-holding capacity. I have compiled two lists of vegetables based on a formula whereby the caloric value was multiplied by the carbohydrate content, then divided by the amount of soluble fiber in each vegetable. The most desirable vegetables are listed first. Those that retain water in the *intestine* may be preferred over those that do not hold water. The "starter" vegetables should be the first dish at lunch and dinner. Starters produce a gel in the stomach and intestines that slows the transit and decreases the fat absorption of the dish you eat next. Eat plenty of starter vegetables until you feel full.

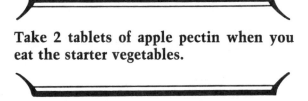

Take 2 tablets of apple pectin when you eat the starter vegetables.

The soluble-fiber properties of the vegetables on the "filler" list are not completely known. Fillers should be the second part of your meal when you need a lot of food to be satisfied. Starters can be used as the second dish too. Do not use fillers to begin a meal. Eat these vegetables raw or steam or bake them. Do not fry. Lemon juice, vinegar, low-caloric dressing, imitation butter, and spices can be used for extra flavoring. Do not add oil or butter.

By beginning with these starters and fillers, you have to do a lot of chewing and so ingest only small amounts of calories just when you are inclined to eat fastest. When you have slowed down (only after full satiation with vegetables), you can eat starches and proteins.

You can mix several vegetables, but don't do it too often because it might increase the amount of food you consume. Avoid any cues that might trigger additional eating. Remember that variety of flavor and color stimulates other senses. It is best to have one kind of vegetable first, such as a lettuce salad, then have another, such as steamed asparagus. Don't tempt yourself with too much choice.

Starter Vegetables

Values: $\dfrac{\text{Cal} \times \text{CHO}}{\text{Soluble Fiber}}$

Zucchini	43
Cucumber	73
Lettuce	83
Broccoli	85
Celery*	94
Summer squash	108
Radish	141
Carrots*	143
Cabbage	144
Turnips	198
Eggplant*	204
Kale	216
Green beans*	284
Beets	288
Asparagus*	399
Cauliflower*	432
Brussel sprouts	436
Tomatoes*	446
Bean sprouts	499
Rutabaga	508

*High water-holding capacity.

Filler Vegetables

Values: $\dfrac{\text{Cal} \times \text{CHO}}{\text{Soluble Fiber}}$

Seaweed	0
Rhubarb	430
Chicory	793
Watercress	948
Artichoke	950
Endive (escarole)	1,264
Kohlrabi	1,326
Olives	1,400
Spinach	1,500
Mustard greens	1,504
Sweet pepper	1,760
Pumpkin	2,241
Fennel	2,596
Mushrooms	3,135
Pimiento	3,272
Hot peppers	3,444

MEATS AND OTHER PROTEINS

Protein intake is optional at breakfast and lunch but is essential at dinner. The proteins listed on page 51 have been selected for their low fat content. Four ounces of protein—the size of a hamburger patty—are allowed at lunch and dinner. Equal quantities of any of these are interchangeable. Always trim away fat and remove poultry skin. If you skip proteins at lunch, you can increase your protein intake at dinner to 8 ounces.

Proteins gradually increase glucagon and CCK levels in your blood and do not disturb your overnight fasting chemistry, so you can have a small amount (1 ounce) at breakfast. Eat 1 thin slice of cheese or ham, fish, or meat, 1 tablespoon of peanut butter, 2 tablespoons of cottage cheese or plain yogurt, or 1 egg any style.

For lunch and dinner, proteins should be eaten after vegetables or fruit to decrease the absorption of the fat they contain.

Proteins have a lasting satiation effect that carries you through between meals without desiring snacks. To obtain full protein benefits, always have them as the last dish of a meal. You can broil, bake, or boil your proteins; frying is allowed only two times a week. Spices can be freely used when preparing proteins. Mustard, lemon juice, and imitation butter are allowed, but catsup is forbidden.

Recommended Proteins

Four-ounce portions (hamburger-patty size) of meat and cheese allowed per main meal; 1-ounce portions (1 slice) at breakfast. Trim fat from meat and remove skin and giblets from poultry.

BEEF	PORK	LAMB	POULTRY	FISH AND SHELLFISH
London broil, flank steak, ground beef, heart, round steak, chuck roast, chuck steak, liver, tongue	None	Loin chops, shoulder, leg	All	All

(Table continued on next page)

Veal and Rabbit	Cheese and Peanut Butter	Cold Cuts	Eggs	Milk
All	Low-fat cottage cheese, 1 thin slice of any cheese, 1 tablespoon peanut butter	Cured ham, boiled ham, meatloaf	All (2 eggs = 4 oz.)	Skim, low-fat, 2 tablespoons plain skim yogurt

SOURCES: *Nutritive Value of American Food* #456 and *Composition of Food* #8 from the Department of Agriculture.

Allowed Spices, Sauces, and Dressings

All spices
Lime
Lemon
Vinegar
Safflower, sunflower, or corn oil for frying.
    Do not add to salads or cooked vegetables.
Tomato sauce without meat
Red peppers
Tabasco
Garlic
Anchovies
Mustard
White clam sauce
Imitation butter (e.g., Butter Buds)
Low-calorie diet dressings

    All other sauces and gravies are *not allowed*.

> Do not eat red meat with any starches such as rice, potatoes, noodles, or macaronis. The combination is high in calories and increases your appetite.

THE BEST FRUITS

The fruits listed below were selected using the same formula as the vegetables: The caloric value was multiplied by the carbohydrate content, then divided by the amount of soluble fiber. Fruits with the lowest figures were chosen for the Bio-Diet. Their water-holding capacity was also taken into consideration.

Selected fruits are allowed on work weeks only at breakfast. On break weeks they are allowed in two out of three meals. They can be eaten raw or dried without added sugar. Cooked fruits are not allowed. All fruit juices except grapefruit, lime, and lemon should be avoided. Fruits can be eaten in place of the starter vegetables to benefit from their soluble-fiber gel property.

Fruit Starters

Values: $\dfrac{\text{Cal} \times \text{CHO}}{\text{Soluble Fiber}}$

Tangerine	345
Orange*	367
Strawberry (3 whole large)	370
Apple*	380
Grapefruit	456
Peach	497
Apricot	652
Cantaloupe half	733

*High water-holding capacity

Fruit starters are to be used instead of vegetable starters *only on break weeks*. Fruits can be fresh or dried.

FOOD PREPARATION SUMMARY

	Don'ts	*Do's*
Starter and filler vegetables	No boiling or frying	Raw, steam, bake
Starches	No frying	Boil, bake, steam
Proteins	All preparation methods are allowed, but frying is limited to twice a week.	
Fruits	Do not cook	Raw or dried

The No-Choice Bio-Diet

The key to some recent successful diets has been the no-choice rule, according to which you must eat, meal by meal, only what is specifically allowed. For those who like the no-choice approach to dieting, I have provided four weekly menus for two work weeks and two break weeks. Some flexibility is allowed on Sunday, if you stay within the boundaries of foods permitted that week. You can do two consecutive work weeks for faster weight loss, but do not combine two break weeks in a row. The best approach to the no-choice Bio-Diet is one work week (#1), one break week (#2), one work week (#3), one break week (#4). After four weeks, repeat the cycle again or follow the flexible, nonspecified Bio-Diet. Bypass break weeks to lose weight faster, provided your doctor allows you to do so.

Weekly Diets

WEEK #1

Work-Week Diet

(For quantities and portions, see pages 43–45.)

BREAKFAST	LUNCH	DINNER
MONDAY Coffee or tea (black or with skim milk) ½ grapefruit 1 slice smoked or pickled fish	Consommé Lettuce salad 1 (3.5-ounce) can water-packed tuna	Clam juice Baked zucchini Spinach salad Roast leg of lamb
TUESDAY Coffee or tea (black or with skim milk) 1 slice Swiss cheese	Diet gelatin Cucumber salad Broiled filet of sole	Diet soda Baked eggplant Watercress salad Roast fowl
WEDNESDAY Coffee or tea (black or with skim milk) 3 strawberries 2 tablespoons plain yogurt	Beef broth Baked summer squash Meatloaf	Consommé madrilene Raw celery, olives, and mushrooms Fried fish

BREAKFAST	LUNCH	DINNER
THURSDAY Coffee or tea (black or with skim milk) 1 slice ham	Grapefruit juice Cole slaw Broiled hamburger	Bouillon Tomato salad Baked carrots Liver or tongue
FRIDAY Coffee or tea (black or with skim milk) 1 egg (any style)	Diet soda Steamed broccoli Deep-fried veal cutlet	Tomato juice Lettuce salad Steamed artichokes Broiled seafood
SATURDAY Coffee or tea (black or with skim milk) 1 apple 2 tablespoons cottage cheese	Vegetable or tomato juice Raw carrots Broiled chicken	Broth Steamed cauliflower Endive and fennel salad Flank steak

SUNDAY

Any combination of favorite foods in prescribed order from work-week menus.

WEEK #2

Break-Week Diet

(For quantities and portions, see pages 45–46.)

BREAKFAST	LUNCH	DINNER
MONDAY Coffee or tea (black or with skim milk) 1 orange 1 egg (any style)	Beef broth Watercress salad Spaghetti with imitation butter or low-calorie margarine	Vegetable or tomato juice Eggplant Raw carrots Chuck steak
TUESDAY Coffee or tea (black or with skim milk) 1 slice ham	Grapefruit juice Asparagus Smoked or pickled fish with lettuce	Diet soda Orange sections Baked carrots Boiled potato Broiled shrimp
WEDNESDAY Coffee or tea (black or with skim milk) 1 peach 1 slice Swiss cheese	Vegetable or tomato juice Cucumber salad Omelet with green peppers	Iced coffee or tea with lemon Steamed zucchini Escarole Veal roast

BREAKFAST	LUNCH	DINNER
THURSDAY Coffee or tea (black or with skim milk) 2 tablespoons cottage cheese	Diet soda Bean sprouts London broil	Clam juice Baked squash Baked potato Roast fowl Candied orange peels
FRIDAY Coffee or tea (black or with skim milk) 1 apple 1 tablespoon peanut butter	Consommé Celery sticks Sliced turkey	Broth ½ grapefruit Green beans Rice Broiled flounder
SATURDAY Coffee or tea (black or with skim milk) 2 tablespoons plain yogurt	Diet gelatin Lettuce salad Fettuccine with clam or tomato sauce	Bouillon 3 large fresh strawberries Tomato salad Broiled beef

SUNDAY

Any combination of favorite foods in prescribed order from break-week menus.

WEEK #3

Work-Week Diet

BREAKFAST	LUNCH	DINNER
MONDAY Coffee or tea (black or with skim milk) 1 orange 2 tablespoons cottage cheese	Vegetable or tomato juice Green beans Broiled hamburger	Consommé Sliced beets Escarole Cod steak
TUESDAY Coffee or tea (black or with skim milk) 1 slice ham	Consommé Lettuce hearts 1 (3.5-ounce) can water-packed tuna	Seltzer with lemon Cucumbers Steamed artichoke Broiled liver
WEDNESDAY Coffee or tea (black or with skim milk) 1 apricot 1 tablespoon peanut butter	Beef broth julienne carrots Baked chicken	Grapefruit juice Baked eggplant Watercress Fried veal cutlet

BREAKFAST	LUNCH	DINNER
THURSDAY Coffee or tea (black or with skim milk) 2 tablespoons plain yogurt	Diet soda Cole slaw Baked ham	Bouillon Steamed turnips Pickled beets London broil
FRIDAY Coffee or tea (black or with skim milk) 3 strawberries 1 slice smoked fish	Club soda with lemon Tomatoes Broiled fish filet	Clam juice Zucchini Chicory salad Roast leg of lamb
SATURDAY Coffee or tea (black or with skim milk) 1 egg (any style)	Bouillon Steamed cabbage Chuck steak	Consommé Broccoli Fennel salad Broiled shrimp

SUNDAY

Any combination of favorite foods in prescribed order from work-week menus.

WEEK #4

Break-Week Diet

BREAKFAST	LUNCH	DINNER
MONDAY Coffee or tea (black or with skim milk) 3 dried apple slices 2 tablespoons plain yogurt	Beef broth Celery sticks Watercress Meatloaf	Iced tea Orange wedges Spinach salad White rice Roast chicken
TUESDAY Coffee or tea (black or with skim milk) Grapefruit juice 1 slice American cheese	Diet soda 1 apple Green salad Fried chicken	Consommé Lettuce Sweet peppers Linguine with margarine or tomato sauce Broiled fish
WEDNESDAY Coffee or tea (black or with skim milk) 1 egg (any style)	Bouillon Cucumbers Escarole Boiled potato Dark or white sliced turkey	Diet gelatin Apple wedges Lettuce and tomato salad Flank steak Candied orange peel

BREAKFAST	LUNCH	DINNER
THURSDAY Coffee or tea (black or with skim milk) 1 apricot 1 slice pickled herring	Iced coffee Orange Brussels sprouts Wild rice Omelet fine herbs	Mineral water with lemon Baked zucchini Spinach Baked potato Roast chicken
FRIDAY Coffee or tea (black or with skim milk) 1 tablespoon peanut butter	Tea with lemon Unsweetened fresh fruit salad Endive salad Spaghetti with clam sauce	Beef broth ½ grapefruit Carrot sticks Asparagus tips Liver
SATURDAY Coffee or tea (black or with skim milk) 2 tablespoons cottage cheese	Diet soda Melon slice Sour relish Broiled hamburger	Vegetable or tomato juice 3 large fresh strawberries Fennel 3 large olives Lamb chops Candied grapefruit peel

SUNDAY
Any combination of favorite foods in prescribed order from break-week menus.

4
Questions I Have Been Asked by My Patients

Q: How many pounds will I lose per week on the Bio-Diet?

A: This is a question everyone asks, but unfortunately I can't answer it for everyone. How rapidly you lose weight depends on several factors. First, your degree of overweight. Obese persons lose more pounds per week than mild overweights. Your age and your sex also have a bearing: Younger people lose weight faster than older ones, and men lose faster than women. The amount and intensity of activities is another consideration, and faithful followers of my exercise program will shed pounds much more quickly than nonexercisers. Finally, if your body chemistry has been disrupted for a long period of time, or you disrupt it by reverting to old eating habits, this will adversely influence the rate of weight loss. So most important is how strictly you follow the diet. Cheaters lose slowly.

To state a figure of weekly weight loss without considering the above factors is misleading. All I can tell you is that you will lose considerable pounds and inches.

TIP FOR WOMEN

Keep a weekly record of your waist, hip, and thigh measurements. Some weeks you may lose more inches than pounds, especially when you are premenstrual.

Q: Are chef's salads permitted on the Bio-Diet?

A: Chef's salads can be eaten if you eat the vegetables first, and then finish with the proteins. Request lemon or vinegar instead of any dressing.

Q: What kinds of omelets can I eat?

A: Plain omelets or with fines herbes can be considered as plain protein.

Q: My largest meal is breakfast. What can I do?

A: Consider your breakfast the dinner meal and eat everything allowed. At lunch, have a small meal such as indicated for breakfast, or have your smallest meal at night.

Q: Can I eat less at lunch and have a snack?

A: I don't allow snacks because it has been documented that two-thirds of all snacks are eaten with either little or no hunger. Try to avoid snacks. Snacking is a bad habit that should be broken. You can drink a caloric fluid (page 47) if you feel ravenously hungry. Take safflower oil capsules when needed for extreme hunger. The combination of an acidic juice and safflower oil capsules gives the best satiation effect.

Q: What kinds of starches are allowed?

A: Brown, wild, and white rice; potatoes; and noodles and macaronis without fillings are allowed on this diet for their low cost, easy availability, and high psychological rewarding value. Brown rice is preferred to polished white rice because it is harder to digest and isn't absorbed as much. Wild rice is even better, but it is extremely expensive.

Q: How can I cook them?

A: Boiling, steaming, or microwave cooking are the best. Baking is only a fair choice. Frying is not allowed.

Q: When can I eat starches?

A: *Only on break weeks.* Have them after a starter dish of vegetables or fruit and a second dish of filler vegetables. Eat starches only after you are satiated with vegetables.

Q: How do you feel about the low-carbohydrate diet?

A: The controversy about low-carbohydrate diets continues. Most research indicates that you lose as much on a low-carbohydrate diet as you do on a carbohydrate-balanced one. The low-carbohydrate diet increases urine output during the first days, which translates into an immediate weight loss. In the long run, the water is recovered and the weight returns. If your kidneys are impaired by disease or age, urea—the final metabolic product of protein—can accumulate in blood and produce toxic effects.

The Bio-Diet is low in carbohydrates on the work weeks and balanced on the break weeks. You will not tax your kidneys or be dehydrated, and you will see a steady loss of weight and/or inches.

Q: How can I tell if I am drinking enough water?

A: On my program you will lose large amounts of water due to sweating during the exercise period. It is important that you replenish your body as soon as possible. The color of your urine is an indication of the degree of concentration of fluids in your body. If it is very dark yellow, you are not getting enough fluids. Your urine should always be light yellow to whitish.

Q: What about high-protein diets?

A: When animals on a high-protein diet are given a low-protein regimen, their eating increases and they gain weight. You might have experienced this weight gain when you went onto a maintenance diet after being on a high-protein plan for several weeks. With the Bio-Diet, this problem doesn't occur because the diet is composed of moderate quantities of protein and has adequate carbohydrates. If you follow this plan your body chemistry will change and your hunger will stay under control.

Q: What about intestinal gas and high-fiber foods?

A: My diet and high-roughage diets have few points in common because I have avoided too much hard vegetable roughage. This type of fiber is poorly tolerated because your intestine can't digest it, causing most people to bloat.

I recommend eating fruits and vegetables with large amounts of 100-percent-digestible soluble fiber. Hard roughage increases stool weight and speeds up transit through the large intestine, while soluble fiber slows the transit of food in the stomach and small intestine and curbs your appetite.

Soluble fiber must be eaten before any meats or starches. Soluble fiber forms a gel in the stomach and intestines, which decreases fat and starch absorption. Part of the starches in noodles and the fats in meat will be eliminated as body waste. Eating vegetables and fruits with lots of soluble fiber as the first dish of a meal is smart dieting.

Q: Why do you decrease solid fat intake while some diets provide for a high fat intake?

A: A high-fat diet increases your CCK, but the excessive use of fat for that purpose might result in high caloric intake and subsequent weight gain as well as arteriosclerosis. I have minimized fat ingestion by selecting foods with low fat content. You should trim excess fat from any meats. I do recommend that you take a small amount of oil 20 minutes before a meal to increase CCK. Add a few drops of oil to your broth or bouillon or take 1 or 2 safflower oil capsules.

Do you remember that liquid oil and proteins or a mixture of the two will decrease subsequent meal intake? The caloric fluids I allow contain just enough fat to release CCK, but not an excess, which would increase adipose tissue.

Q: What seasonings can I use with starches?

A: At serving time, you can add the sauces and spices listed on page 52, a small amount of grated low-fat mozzarella or romano cheese, margarine, or imitation butter.

Q: What proteins can be eaten with starches?

A: Poultry, fish, and shellfish are the only proteins that can be eaten with starches.

Q: Do you have any recipes for starches?

A: The Bio-Diet is a flexible set of rules that can be applied to common foods. It will modify your present biochemistry as much as possible to achieve your weight goal. I'm not trying to improve your cooking skills. As long as you stay within the Bio-Diet framework you can cook anything and everything!

Q: Should potatoes be cooked with or without the skins?

A: I favor the cooking of potatoes with their skins to keep their water-holding capacity intact. However, you can eat them any way you like except fried. Remember that potato chips are fried.

Q: **Why can't I have cereal at breakfast?**

A: Most ready-to-eat cereals are sugar-coated and provide unwanted calories. Even the few sugar-free cereals are carbohydrates, which are not allowed in the mornings. Although some cereals contain large amounts of roughage, soluble fiber in the best of them—except oat bran—ranges from 4 to 21 percent, while fruits and vegetables contain from 19 to 60 percent. If, on occasion, you do eat carbohydrates in the morning, you would be better off eating fruit than cereal.

Q: **Can I have a snack before going to bed?**

A: Eating before going to bed shortens the effect of overnight fasting and reduces fat breakdown. You can drink a low-calorie fluid, but you should not eat at bedtime.

Q: **Can I have diet desserts?**

A: When you have reached your weight loss goal, you can have a small portion of a regular dessert. Meantime, enjoy fruits and candied fruit peels on break weeks. Have dietetic gelatin as a last resort.

Q: **Can I use two starter vegetables instead of one starter and one filler?**

A: Yes. Starters can be the second dish of a meal instead of a filler. The Thursday dinner of the Week #1 sample diet is an example of a starter as a second dish.

Q: **I can't eat vegetables. How can I still follow your diet?**

A: First, follow the caloric fluids rule. Then have allowed fruits instead of vegetables. As a last resort, buy apple pectin tablets and have 2 or 3 tablets before solid food intake. *Warning:* If you do not eat fruits and vegetables, you are not getting a balanced diet.

Q: May I eat one fruit and then a starter or filler vegetable?

A: Yes, fruits can be a first dish, and a starter or filler vegetable can be the second dish. Fillers should always be a second dish. Fruits can be the second dish on break weeks.

Q: Can I eat double amounts (about 8 ounces) of protein at dinner if I have passed it up at lunch?

A: Yes, but it is better to have protein intake spread out in small amounts at breakfast, lunch, and dinner.

Q: Why is milk not allowed on the list of caloric fluids that curb the appetite?

A: Milk does not curb the appetite, probably because it is alkaline and neutralizes stomach juices. You are allowed skim milk at breakfast and with coffee or tea at any time.

Q: Can I have yogurt?

A: Yes, you can have plain yogurt made from skimmed milk. If you like flavor, add cinnamon, saccharin, diet jelly, or allowed fruits (fresh or dried). You cannot eat flavored yogurt because it contains sugar or fruit preserves. Unsweetened plain yogurt can be eaten for breakfast, lunch, or dinner. Two tablespoons is enough for breakfast and 1 cup is allowed at lunch or dinner. Yogurt is a protein, so a vegetable or a fruit starter must precede yogurt ingestion at lunch or dinner.

Q: Why do you advise eating dried fruits? Aren't they high in sugar and calories?

A: Dried fruits have the same amount of sugar and fiber as fresh fruit, but less water. They seem to be high in carbohydrates and calories, but after taking their lack of moisture into consideration the actual composition of dried fruits is close to fresh fruits. Dried fruits provide a satisfactory sweet taste in the mouth and a concentrated gel of soluble fiber in the stomach. The drawback is that some dried fruits have potassium sorbate and other preservatives added. Check the package, or buy from a health food store.

Q: **Why is peanut butter permitted at breakfast?**

A: Peanut butter is low in carbohydrates when made without sugar (check the label) and is high in protein, vegetable fat, and fiber. It has a high satiation value. No bread or jelly is allowed. One tablespoon of peanut butter has 94 calories, which can keep you going without eating for several hours.

Q: **Do I get all the U.S. Recommended Daily Allowances (USRDA) of nutrients when following the Bio-Diet?**

A: Absolutely. The Bio-Diet meets all USRDA for proteins, vitamins, and minerals. It supplies proteins of the highest biological value; those that contain all the indispensable amino acids in balanced quantities.

Q: **I can't help it—I go on pizza and ice cream binges. How can I slow down absorption? (P.S., I hate fruits and vegetables.)**

A: You are a tough one! When you feel a binge coming on, swallow 2 tablets of apple pectin, 2 capsules of safflower oil, and 1 tablet of tryptophane, then drink a glass of grapefruit juice, water, or diet soda. Do some exercise. Your binge will then probably be a short one.

Q: **I do not lose as much weight during break weeks as I do during work weeks. What should I do?**

A: It is normal to show lower weight loss during break weeks than during work weeks. Break weeks will break down as much fat as work weeks, but it might not show on the scale because of water retention. This might happen to people who retain water when they eat carbohydrates. Avoid salt to reduce water retention during break weeks.

Don't become discouraged during break weeks. Try the work diet for two weeks to see a greater weight loss, then go back to the normal cycle.

Q: Am I going to be hungry during break weeks?

A: You will not feel hungry at all after the first forty-eight hours on the Bio-Diet, and this effect is sustained all along during break and work weeks. People who are going through a period of excessive stress and are unable to relax with the relaxation reflex might have difficulties following the diet. The same holds true for alcoholics. Patients have told me that on the occasions when they have wanted forbidden food, the desire has disappeared after drinking one of the caloric drinks on page 47. One or 2 capsules of safflower oil helps too.

Q: Can I eat sandwiches?

A: Open sandwiches made with allowed protein foods are okay only after you have reached your goal. Regular sandwiches are not on my diet. Two slices of whole wheat bread provide 134 calories. If you prefer white bread, count on 152 calories. Buttered bread brings your calorie count up to 250 calories. Add 132 calories from 2 slices of ham and 60 calories from 1 slice of dietetic cheese—more than 442 calories in one small ham and cheese sandwich. If mortadella replaces the ham and American cheese is substituted for the dietetic one, your calorie intake jumps up to 510 calories! The satiation value of a sandwich is very low, and you will be hungry soon. But sooner or later you will want to eat a sandwich. Order an unbuttered roll and remove all the soft inside, leaving only the crust. Avoid cold cuts other than ham. In fast food chains, the fish filet or chicken sandwich is your best choice, provided you remove the soft part of the bread. Forget cheese sandwiches and hot heroes altogether.

Q: **Can I eat the trimmed fat and skin I have removed from meat and fowl prior to the meal?**

A: No way! This is solid fat and should not be substituted for safflower capsules. The discarded fat from animals is high in saturated oils that are damaging to your heart. Solid food takes time to be absorbed, so it does not provide immediate satiation. Animal fat should go into the garbage can and not into your stomach!

Q: **Why are whole olives on the diet but nuts not permitted?**

A: Both olives and nuts have high salt content. Seville and green olives are the two varieties I recommend. They are usually eaten before meals, often with other raw vegetables. Discarding olive pits involves some manual steps, which increase awareness of the eating process, and the discarded pits are a reminder of how many have been consumed. The total calorie content of 1 pound of pitted olives varies between 442 and 526 calories. The fat content is approximately 58 grams.

But nuts are grabbed before meals and swallowed in combination with an alcoholic drink. They are usually unshelled, which makes them easy to eat. A pound of peanuts contains a whopping 2,654 calories and has a high fat content of 226 grams.

So you see that you can save more than 2,000 calories per pound of food if you eat olives instead of nuts.

Q: Can I pass up breakfast altogether?

A: Yes, you can if you have always skipped it before, but if you like to snack in the late morning, it is better to have a small breakfast to break that habit.

Q: What about skipping lunch?

A: *You cannot skip lunch if you skipped breakfast!* You can bypass lunch if you have had breakfast. If you snack before dinner or while preparing it, meal skipping is not allowed. Persons suffering from hypoglycemia, diabetes, anemia, and cardiovascular disorders should eat all of the allowed meals.

Q: Do you recommend any pasta?

A: Any pasta without cheese or meat filling is permitted. If you choose bulky pastas, such as twist macaroni, you can save calories. One cup of twist macaroni weighs 84 grams versus 134 grams/cup for spiral macaroni.

Q: Is there any difference in the number of calories contained in fresh home-cooked vegetables and in canned ones?

A: Home-cooked fruits and vegetables have more volume, more vitamins, and fewer calories than canned ones. For example: One cup of fresh asparagus spears weighs 145 grams and yields 29 calories, while 1 cup of canned spears weighs 235 grams and has 47 calories. You save 40 percent of the calories by buying and cooking fresh foods.

Q: Do I have to eat all my breakfast, lunch, and dinner or may I skip food when I'm not feeling hungry?

A: This diet provides a list of allowed foods, rules on eating, and limits on maximum intake. *It does not force you to eat all of what is offered.* Many of my patients eat half of what is on the diet and feel great while losing fat. If you wish to reduce the quantity of food intake, proceed as follows: Once you have finished the first vegetable, ask, "Am I hungry?" If you do not feel hungry, stop eating and leave the table. If your answer is yes, continue with a filler vegetable or eat more of the starter vegetables and repeat the question "Am I hungry?" And so on. Do not stop if you feel you are still hungry, because you will try to fill that hunger later by snacking on the wrong food. Skip the starches or proteins or both if you are going to skip anything.

Q: What **can** I eat at a party?

A: As a general rule of thumb, follow the same dietary guidelines you have learned. First, drink fluids, broth, soup, juice, tea or coffee; follow with fiber foods until satiated; finish with proteins. Have few starches and no sugars.

Plan ahead and stick to it. For an evening party, moderate your food intake by having a late lunch and skipping dinner. Just before leaving for the party, have coffee with skim milk, bouillon, vegetable or tomato juice, diet gelatin, soup, or 2 capsules of safflower oil with grapefruit, lemon, or lime juice. At the party, drink a diet soda, mineral water, or club soda followed by a few olives, mushrooms, or any available green vegetable. Avoid the dips and forget all the nuts and snack foods. Later on, you can eat a little ham, roast beef, or chicken. Avoid starches, potato salads, and bread. Drink coffee or diet soda and avoid tempting desserts and alcohol. If you want to have a drink, get it near the end of the party, not when it is just starting, because alcohol can destroy your motivation. If fruits are available, have one piece. Stay closer to a workweek diet than a break-week diet.

PARTY-GOING

1. Don't stay home instead of going out—that increases depression and eating.
2. Don't have dinner before the party—you might end up eating twice.
3. Don't isolate yourself—that increases postparty gorging.
4. Don't stay near the food.
5. Don't refuse to dance due to shyness. Dancing is a good aerobic exercise that curbs appetite and breaks down fat.

Remember, have fun, not food!

Q: What alcohol can I drink?

A: No alcohol is allowed on my diet. Since there are always rule breakers, the following might help regarding booze intake:

Alcoholic drinks do not quench your thirst. If you are thirsty, have a nonalcoholic fluid (water, grapefruit, lemon, or lime juice, diet soda), then enjoy one light alcoholic drink. Drink a small glass of brandy, red wine, cognac, or sherry at room temperature. Cold drinks numb your taste buds and make it easy to overdrink. Start your meals with nonalcoholic fluids and open wine for the main course. You will drink less and feel better.

Drinking alcohol before or between meals will increase your insulin and sugar levels. This in turn activates your appetite, an unwanted effect.

Q: Why do you allow shellfish on your diet? Isn't shellfish high in cholesterol?

A: Shellfish, eggs, and some meats are all high in cholesterol, but they are excellent sources of proteins. There is no perfect food (except mother's milk for babies), and I feel that the variety of foods balances the drawbacks of each. If you follow my diet, your total cholesterol intake will be lower than the cholesterol intake of the average American diet.

Q: Can I have peanut butter and jelly sandwiches?

A: Once you have reached your ideal weight and shape, and if you continue to exercise and eat prudently, you will be able to eat almost anything. Athletes and dancers eat all kinds of junk food and stay slim because they have good cardiovascular and muscular systems, which keep their body chemistries in good order.

Q: Should I take vitamin and mineral supplements?

A: Minerals are essential for body building and burning fat. Some minerals present in food in very small amounts are called trace elements. They increase the speed of metabolism, but the daily need for some of them is not known. If you follow the Bio-Diet, you will obtain all the trace elements necessary for a healthy body. If you eat less than what I recommend, you might need supplementation. Be sure that your vitamin pill includes minerals.

My diet provides all the recommended daily allowances of vitamins. However, since you may try to overdo it or do not follow the diet too closely, I recommend a multiple vitamin supplement. If you are a heavy smoker, a social drinker, or have recently had the flu, you might have a deficiency in some specific vitamin, which the supplement would help replenish.

When you are changing your eating habits, you should supplement vitamins and minerals.

Q: **Is there a link between my sex life and my weight problem?**

A: No matter how your sex life is, weight loss can improve it, because weight reduction corrects many of the psychological and chemical abnormalities that infringe on your sexual urge. Your true motivation to lose weight is probably sexual. This might be expressed as "I want to dress fashionably," "have my clothes fit better," "look younger," "wear a bathing suit." You don't explicitly say that you want to dress fashionably to attract a mate, have your clothes fit better to look sexy, look younger to appeal to younger, more active people, or be able to wear a bathing suit to call attention to your body.

While sex influences your motivation to lose weight, fat distribution plays a role in your behavior. The link between sexual behavior and fat is very strong in women. Women tend to gain weight in areas of sexual significance, whereas men do not. An increase in the size of the breasts or buttocks can produce anxiety about body shape. This unwanted anxiety results in excessive self-consciousness, which can interfere with sexual intimacy.

Don't despair; there is hope. It is not confirmed that fat is an unconscious defense against sex. In fact, some studies have shown that overweight women do not avoid sex. In a study comparing the sexual habits of overweight and slim couples, it was found that the heavier group had sex as often as the others and the women had a higher orgasm rate. The latter might be due to a higher level of all sexual hormones. Heavier women endure more menstrual irregularities than other women, but dieting regularizes their periods.

Overweight menopausal women have excessive

amounts of sexual hormones. This has two benefits: a reduction of breast atrophy and an absence of facial wrinkles. But among the problems with excessive amounts of sexual hormones are increased menstrual disturbances and more fat deposits. Remember that sexual hormones are injected into beef cattle to increase their weight before slaughter. Birth-control pills have the same effect on you as hormone injections have on animals. The increased hormones disturb your unbalanced carbohydrate metabolism by increasing the insulin level, which interferes with weight loss.

Dr. Victor Wynn observed that birth-control pills change a normal metabolism to that of an obese woman and alter the metabolism of an obese woman to that of a diabetic. Between 50 and 75 percent of diabetics are overweight. Impotence in an overweight man is frequently the reason he seeks medical help and discovers that he has diabetes.

Q: What is the effect of this diet on my heart?

A: My program is good for your heart. By following it, you will decrease certain health risks.

There are three laboratory tests that evaluate the likelihood of a heart attack or stroke: the blood cholesterol levels, the triglyceride levels, and the high-density lipoprotein-C levels (HDL-C). High levels of cholesterol and triglycerides and low HDL-C readings are linked with arteriosclerosis, the fattening, narrowing, and hardening of the arteries. Coronary heart disease is a result of arteriosclerosis and accounts for 1.2 million heart attacks every year in the United States.

The ideal cholesterol level is between 170 and 180 milligrams per deciliter of blood, but you are probably safe if you register less than 200 mg/dl. To reach this level, you must decrease your cholesterol intake. How can you do it? Just follow the Bio-Diet, because it is low in cholesterol.

Mrs. H., seventy, lost 15 pounds following the Bio-Diet and her cholesterol count went from 372 mg/dl to 272 mg/dl in less than a month.

If you are overweight, you more than likely have an increased concentration in the blood of triglycerides. Triglyceride levels should be less than 120 mg/dl. Several studies strongly link an increase in blood triglyceride levels to coronary heart disease.

My program helps decrease triglycerides because it produces weight loss, is low in cholesterol, and reduces the consumption of sugar and saturated fats. This combination of factors will effectively reduce triglycerides to help your heart beat longer.

Mrs. H., mentioned above, had a triglyceride level that decreased from 343 mg/dl to 141 mg/dl in the same period.

The high-density lypoprotein-C (HDL-C) level is a more precise indicator of your heart attack risk than cholesterol and triglyceral levels. The more HDL-C in your blood, the more likely you will *not* have a heart attack. Why? Because HDL-C acts as a scavenger that picks up cholesterol from the tissues and carries it to the liver for destruction. It might also help break down fat. A healthy HDL-C level is more than 65 mg/dl. The exercise program in Chapter 5 will help decrease your weight, reduce your measurements in targeted areas, and increase your HDL-C levels to protect your heart.

Recent research has proved that the arteriosclerotic process that brings about narrowing of the arteries can be prevented, arrested, and reversed. My program has been designed with these objectives in mind. I have considered your heart as well as your stomach. You can have a slim figure as well as good arteries. Work on it!

Q: What are your thoughts on salt?

A: The average American consumes almost 14 pounds of salt a year. There is a strong correlation between high salt intake and high blood pressure. Some eaters of lots of salt develop hypertension, but it is unpredictable who will suffer from it and who won't. If you are overweight, you probably will be vulnerable to hypertension. Salt is not recommended on a regular basis.

My diet has an adequate amount of salt. There is no need for adding salt while cooking or eating. Some readers' doctors might have advised them to restrict their salt intake even more. If so, follow my diet and comply with your doctor's instructions by proceeding as follows:

1. Substitute low-salt or unsalted broth, soups, tomato juice, cottage cheese, margarine, and peanut butter for regular products.
2. Rarely eat ham, Swiss cheese, American-flavor processed dietetic cheese, meatloaf, or olives.
3. Use very little canned meat, poultry, or fish, and avoid salted or pickled fish such as herring, lox, or anchovies.
4. Limit shellfish to three times a week.
5. Avoid baking soda or powder; prepared salad dressings; horseradish; celery, onion, or garlic salts; meat tenderizer (MSG); tomato paste; and pickled relish.
6. Read labels before you buy and do not use products that include soda, sodium, NA, sodium sulfite, or are packed in brine or salt.

High-Salt Foods

Canned vegetables
Cheese
Corned beef
Fresh kale
Olives
Mayonnaise
Potato chips
Pretzels
Sauerkraut
Soda crackers
Tomato catsup
Breakfast cereals
Hot dogs and cold cuts
Nuts

Q: Are cookies, cakes, ice cream, pizza, bread, and so on forbidden forever?

A: Not at all. You will be able to enjoy them once your chemistry has changed to the point that your insulin remains stable and your sugar tolerance improves. According to your degree of overweight, it will take at least three months of dieting and exercise before you will be ready to eat these goodies and not gain weight.

5
Exercise

Recipe for Living Longer

According to recent figures from the Department of Agriculture, Americans now eat 10–15 percent fewer calories than in 1965–66, but our body weight has remained stable because of a lack of exercise. The average American begins to fatten up and get lazy at about age twenty-five.

Animal studies indicate longevity is increased with exercise. This has been confirmed in humans also. In 1979, the American Cancer Society released a twenty-year study of one million people. Death rates were considerably higher among people who did not exercise at all, and the rate decreased as the amount of exercise increased.

A study conducted at Washington University in Saint Louis shows that the exercised heart beats better. Geriatric runners had only 4 percent decline in cardiovascular efficiency due to age, but sedentary senior citizens had an 8 percent decline. Exercise lowers cholesterol in the blood but increases HDL-C, which protects against coronary heart disease. Exercise is no guarantee against heart attacks, but if you do have one, a good cardiovascular system means you will have more chance of surviving it!

How Exercise Works

Exercise helps decrease fat; inactivity promotes fattening. Exercise helps by several mechanisms:

1. Exercise doubles the metabolic rate and keeps it higher for up to twenty-four hours due to the release of the hormone adrenaline.

2. Exercise alleviates depression, tension, and anxiety and gives a feeling of well-being which helps to curb emotional eating. These emotional effects occur because of an increase of serotonin.
3. Exercise increases muscle caloric expenditure ten to twenty times, which helps burn fat deposits.
4. Exercise decreases eating and increases fluid intake. Both actions are good for fat loss.
5. Exercise decreases the excessive insulin output of overweight patients that promotes fat.
6. Exercise improves blood circulation in fat and muscles. Fat will be consumed from those areas of increased circulation if the person is also dieting.
7. Exercise enhances your self-image and provides motivation to continue on a weight-loss program.
8. Trained high-density muscles consume calories primarily from fat; untrained muscles consume mostly glucose.

Walking slowly or performing light calisthenics consumes very few calories. For example, 15 minutes of bending to touch your toes, stretching, and a few calisthenics consumes only 50 calories. This is the equivalent of one cookie . . . and you thought you were exercising! I believe a low level of activity produces fat deposits and overeating is secondary to a weight problem. Remember: Many overweight people do not overeat.

The ability of muscles to contract is what gives them the capacity for movement. When a muscle contracts, it is the total effort of millions of cells. There are two kinds of contractile muscle cells: the slow-twist and the fast-twist.

Slow-twist muscle cells function when long, sustained, slow contractions are required. The slow-twist cells produce the contractions that maintain your body posture, and are involved in slow walking, light calisthenics, and carrying weight. Because they are working continuously, they must be efficient and consume very few calories, otherwise the energy deposits stored in the adipose tissue would be depleted quickly. These muscle cells are like an efficient car with the engine running at low speed—it uses little fuel. Overweight people are pros at working slow-twist cells to consume very few calories.

The fast-twist muscle cells are called into action when a rapid movement is required or when an effort is greater than the slow-twist cells are able to handle. They are able to work rapidly for periods not exceeding 1 minute. Fast-twist muscle cells are not fuel efficient, so they consume lots of calories in a short time. To continue with the car analogy, fast-twist cells are like a car engine speeding up while carrying a heavy passenger load—fuel consumption is phenomenal. *Fast-twist cells are the key to slimness!*

How to Get Your Muscles to Burn More Calories

We all have slow-twist and fast-twist muscle cells, but the proportions of each vary in individuals. Sprinters or other athletes with natural speed capabilities are born with proportionately more fast-twist cells. They can burn enormous amounts of calories in a very short time, whereas endurance runners, such as marathoners, have more slow-twist cells and waste few calories. Sprinters who are also good marathon runners have both cells.

We do not yet know the percentage of fast-twist and slow-twist muscle cells in the overweight, but we do know that overweights burn few calories. It would be to their advantage to change their muscle structure. The number of slow- or fast-twist muscle cells cannot be changed, but the strength of either one as well as the ability to delay fatigue can be altered. By increasing the strength of the fast-twist cells, it is possible to raise the number of calories consumed by the muscles. Fast-twist cell strength grows with frequent exercise. Activities that require the repetition of speedy movements against a light to moderate resistance (such as running and cycling) will increase fast-twist muscle cell strength. Regular exercise four times a week will delay fatigue by increasing the capability of the muscles to release heat and energy. There is also increased muscle density and firmness.

Exercising this type of muscle consumes more calories per minute of work, which allows a shorter exercise period.

Exercise a Lot . . . Diet a Little!

Now the good news: If you continue to exercise when your muscles are firm, you will be able to eat more and not gain weight or else eat less and lose fat much faster.

If you do not have a regular exercise program, you will be doomed to overweight or have fatty hips, thighs, or abdomen. You must make up your mind. If you stick to my exercise program, you will not have to bother dieting after losing your fat.

A Word for Women

Women are often afraid of developing bulky muscles, but studies of children show that boys have more nuclei in their cells than girls. The more nuclei a cell has, the more it can increase in size. Girls are limited in their muscle growth. Large amounts of male hormones also help muscle growth, and women have very tiny amounts of those hormones. Anybody who wants to develop muscles must work at it many hours a day. My exercise program of few minutes of work does not produce bulky muscles at all. Large muscles are made by slow, repetitive movements against heavy resistance, whereas I advise fast movements working with moderate resistance. I am opposed to slow, repetitive weight-lifting movements because they decrease mobilization and utilization of fat and they do not increase the oxygen supply. In my program, the turtle does not win over the hare.

I hope you are now convinced that your muscles can be firm and consume more calories without becoming bulky. By the way, a woman's general muscle strength is about 65 percent that of a man, whereas female chewing muscles have 80 percent the strength of males'.

Fast muscle contractions followed by frequent rest periods will increase your total energy output and use up to 75 percent of the calories you consume. Muscle work will produce local heat and improve the blood flow into the exercised muscles and the surrounding fat. The active adipose tissues will release more fat for combustion than the resting ones. Remember: Maximum spot fat reduction will be achieved *only* if you are dieting. Exercise alone cannot produce significant loss of fat because the fuel supply will come from food instead of your adipose tissue.

There is evidence to suggest that without exercise, mobilization of fat occurs at random. Exercised muscle areas have a higher metabolic rate and greater blood flow.

Exercise is the major factor in losing fat specifically where you want to—it increases localized fat metabolic activity. A Swedish team of doctors recently published a paper proving that short bursts of heavy exercise with frequent rest periods increases utilization of fat as fuel instead of sugar. That is exactly what we want to occur. Exercise will multiply the fat loss produced by a low-caloric diet, and a larger percentage of fat will be consumed from the active areas.

How does the exercise of specific muscles burn the surrounding fat? Muscle contractions produce heat. Heat is released locally and is carried away in the blood. The amount of fuel consumed by muscle contractions depends on the speed of the contractions and the resistance to it. Muscle ability to use calories efficiently is considerably reduced at high speed, resulting in a sharp rise in fuel consumption. Increasing the speed of muscle contractions and the resistance to it—weights—produces even more heat and uses more fuel. To meet those needs there is an increase in blood flow to the muscle to provide oxygen, sugar, and fat fuel. The blood flow to the surrounding fat tissue increases 64 percent above normal resting level. The blood flow into the fat deposits releases hormones that break down fat.

Adrenaline is a hormone that raises the metabolic rate and frees fat from deposits. Exercise raises your adrenaline blood level to five times above the norm. Exercise also activates the enzyme LPL, which breaks down fat. LPL is abundant in exercised muscles and fat; adrenaline comes from the blood. While the muscles work, your adrenaline and LPL will be busy trimming fat.

To check the activity of the exercised area, my patients use a Fever Scan or a Clinitemp, a simple, inexpensive (approximately two dollars) strip of paper that shows the temperature of your skin. It is reusable and can be purchased at your local drugstore. First, check the temperature of your forehead and of the area to be exercised and write them down. After exercising, check the temperature of both areas again. The exercised area should show a rise in temperature. Sometimes only your forehead temperature increases, but that is okay if you have very thick adipose tissue. If there is no increase in either place, it means that you have not exercised enough or have made a mistake in the measurement. The strip should be applied to dry skin. Do not expect a large increase in temperature—1 degree Fahrenheit is sufficient. If the room is too cold, it will block a temperature increase; a too-warm room is dangerous to your health. Exercise in a room at a comfortable temperature. The area to be exercised should not be bare. Wear warm-up clothes or leotards, but avoid plastic exercise clothing.

Losing and Regaining Weight (the Yo-Yo Syndrome)

When activity drops, food intake does not decrease proportionately, so a person gains weight. I have found when I reviewed the charts of certain patients that many who were dieting only had gained back all the weight they had lost, while all those who were successful in keeping their weights down were exercising. Sooner or later, both sedentary and active patients have discontinued their maintenance diets.

These observations confirmed what I have always suspected: Compliance with a diet depends on the reward—weight loss. Maintenance diets are meant to maintain a previously achieved weight loss, but there is no longer any additional reward. Motivation fails because there is no weight loss. Realistically, you have only two choices if you want to stay slim: Either cut down the quantity you eat by following a maintenance diet or use up more calories by exercising.

A maintenance diet is difficult to follow without supervision. Exercise is more satisfying because of the feelings of well-being and sense of achievement that accompany it.

The solution to the "yo-yo" syndrome was provided when it was found that very-low-caloric diets break down muscle mass. Many on-and-off dieting attempts end with muscle destruction, reducing the size and strength of the muscles. When dieting stops, the reduced muscle mass is not enough to keep up with caloric intake, and weight gain follows. Exercise is the only answer. The National Aeronautics and Space Administration (NASA) learned this the hard way. Astronauts in the Skylab program suffered severe muscle destruction. Increasing their caloric intake met with little success, but increasing the intensity of the crew's exercise program solved the problem.

Interval Training Is the Answer

You are going to be surprised if you are resigned to a long, exhausting, boring exercise program. *Excellent results can be obtained in just 9 minutes of work 4 times a week!* How? By working your muscles in 30-second bursts of activity. After relaxing your muscles another 30 seconds, you continue working on and off for 9 minutes. It's so simple and effective! Called "Interval Training," it is the best system to maintain a high level of fat consumption. Interval training is better than continuous exercise because it increases oxygen availability to the muscles and fat, which postpones muscle fatigue and improves their capacity to use fat as fuel.

Muscle contractions consume oxygen, carbohydrates, and fat. At low levels of exercise intensity, muscles consume mostly carbohydrates and very little fat. During moderate levels of exercise activity, fat fuel is preferred over carbohydrates.

The oxygen supply of overweight people is depleted at a lower level of exercise intensity than slim people. This means that the short oxygen supply capacity of overweights curtails the intensity of the exercise and the consumption of fat as fuel. But muscles work without oxygen for only 1 minute; after that, lactic acid (a byproduct of fuel consumption) increases and produces several unwanted effects. It blocks the breakdown of fat in the storage areas and also disturbs the way fat is used as fuel by the muscles. When out-of-condition individuals exercise moderately for more than 1 minute without rest periods, high levels of lactic acid are released. This happens because an untrained cardiovascular system can't supply the blood and the oxygen required by the working muscles. So lactic acid levels rise, fatigue follows, and fat breakdown ends. The obstacles of a short oxygen reserve and the unwanted production of lactic acid would discourage anyone. Another problem is that overweight people have a high level of insulin resistance, which quickly builds up fat. To make things worse, if their eating is high in carbohydrates, blood lactate concentrations are higher both at rest and during exercise. The more carbohydrates there are in the diet, the more those carbohydrates will be burned instead of fat. After meeting with disappointing results, overweights soon drop exercise programs before the training benefits can be discerned. Overweights do have one advantage: Their energy expenditure is 10–50 percent higher per minute of exercise than for their slim counterparts.

Interval training, as opposed to continuous exercise, makes the most of this advantage by producing far less lactic acid. Interval training produces low levels of lactic acid because oxygen can be stored during the rest periods. *Interval training can provide fat loss from the very first day of exercise!* The early results encourage continued motivation to exercise long enough to decrease insulin resistance. Because of the frequent rest periods, you can work out intermittently at very high rates rather comfortably for prolonged periods of time.

Interval training is also excellent for cardiovascular conditioning. You do not have to be an Olympic runner to enjoy the conditioning benefits of interval training. Research has shown that you consume more energy while walking if you change the speed up or down.

Training with Weights versus Weight Lifting

Interval training is an effective way to increase your maximum work capacity and improve your cardiovascular fitness. Slow lifting of heavy weights increases the size of your muscles without improving fitness. Some of the interval training techniques will teach you fast lifting of light weights to increase the natural resistance of your body, help tone muscles, and consume calories.

Do not worry about becoming muscular. An excellent

Canadian report found that working with weights improved women's total body strength, but it did not increase the muscle bulk as it did in men.

Lifting heavy weights increases the size of the slow-twist cells in muscles. These are the cells that burn very few calories. Interval training with light weights firms, trims, and activates the fast-twist cells.

The Exercise Prescription

While trying to lose weight, the exercise prescription is now as important as the drug prescription used to be. My exercise prescription consists of the following:

1. Three minutes of warm-up exercises to get your muscles ready and decrease the risk of injury.
2. Nine minutes of interval training to increase fitness and burn fat.
3. Three minutes of cooling-down activity to ensure a smooth transition and equilibrium between the blood trapped in your muscles and your increased need for oxygen.

The 3-minute warm-up period consists of stretching exercises and light activity such as fast walking, slow cycling, or slow jogging.

The 9-minute interval training consists of alternating walking with jogging; alternating jogging with running; outdoor or indoor cycling; jumping rope; or a special exercise named the D-squat.

The 2-to-3-minute cooling-down period consists of walking, slow cycling, or light calisthenics.

Exercise is limited to 4 times per week on alternate days. I do not advise increasing the frequency of exercises above the specified 4 times a week. The body needs to rest, and several reports indicate that too much exercise often raises the risk of injuries. Practicing sports besides your regular scheduled program is fine, but do not substitute a sport for your exercise program.

The intensity of your exercise during the 9 minutes of interval training depends on the heart rate you achieve while exercising. If your heart beats more than 140 beats per minute, you should slow down. You should increase your efforts when your heart rate drops below 130 beats per minute. To check your pulse, press lightly with the tip of your fingers upon the radial artery in the wrist or the carotid artery in the neck. Take your pulse during the resting phases of your exercise. Resting periods do not mean standing still—just keep moving at a slower pace.

You should be able to complete the 9 minutes of exercise while keeping your pulse at 65–70 beats per 30 seconds. Check your pulse every couple of minutes and try to keep it within prescribed limits. You will notice after three or four weeks of training that the exercises become easier and raising your pulse becomes more difficult. This is great, because you should always work at a steady pulse rate of 65–70 beats per 30 seconds. To do so, just cut the resting time down from 30 to 15 seconds; then if your pulse still does not rise while exercising, increase your speed. After you have obtained the training effect and become fit, you can add heavier weights or resistance to your interval training.

Total Reducing or Spot Reducing

My exercise program consists of warm-up exercises followed by interval training and ending with some cooling-down activity. The interval training is divided into a general part to increase fitness and lose weight and a more specific part to reduce different areas of the body.

The general part must be done first whether you are underweight, slightly overweight, or obese. You can then follow with the specific part provided you are less than 20 pounds overweight. Now look at Table I below to find out your ideal weight.

For example, if you are a 5'4" woman who weighs 150 pounds, Table I indicates your ideal weight is 120 pounds. Now look at Table II (page 101). Because you are more than 20 pounds overweight, you should exercise only with techniques from the general part for the full 9 minutes. As soon as you lose 10 pounds, you should start to use exercises from both the general and specific parts.

Table I: Recommended Weight for Your Height *

HEIGHT	MEN	WOMEN
4'10"	—	102
4'11"	—	104
5'0"	—	107
5'1"	—	110
5'2"	123	113
5'3"	127	116
5'4"	130	120
5'5"	133	123
5'6"	136	128
5'7"	140	132
5'8"	145	136
5'9"	149	140
5'10"	153	144
5'11"	158	148
6'0"	162	152
6'1"	166	—
6'2"	171	—
6'3"	176	—
6'4"	181	—

*Height without shoes, weight without clothes. This is based on the average population and might not be ideal for some. What pleases your eye is best. (Adapted from a table from the Metropolitan Life Insurance Company)

Table II: Interval Training Times

	GENERAL PART Minutes of Exercise	SPECIFIC PART Minutes of Exercise
More than 20 pounds overweight	9	0
0 to 20 pounds overweight	6	3
Underweight	3	6

Warm-ups

Muscular activity should begin with slow warm-up stretching exercises to decrease the possibility of injury. There is no need to check your pulse because these exercises are only preliminary.

Warm-up Exercise #1:

Sit on the floor with your feet placed flat against a wall. *Slowly* stretch extended hands toward toes. Hold for 5 seconds. Repeat 2 more times.

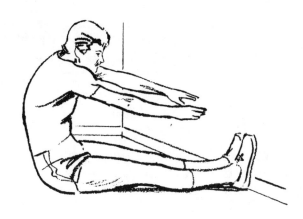

Warm-up Exercise #2:

Stand erect. Bend over toward your toes as far as you can without forcing or bouncing. Hold for a count of 10. Repeat 2 more times.

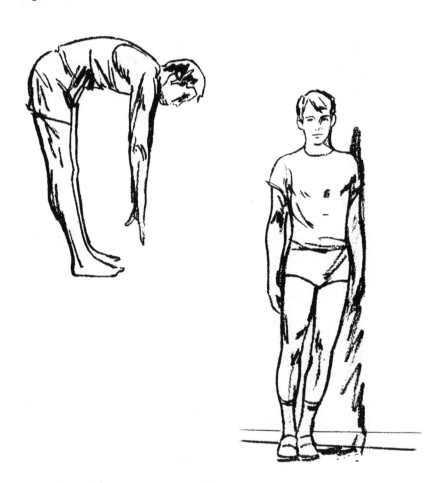

Warm-up Exercise #3:

Stand two feet away from a wall, rest the shoulder against it, and let your hip sag toward it. Hold for a count of 5. Do 3 times on each side.

Exercise

Warm-up Exercise #4:

Lean against a wall with arms outstretched so that your body angles toward it. Keeping your back straight and without lifting the heels, bend elbows and lean toward the wall. Hold for a count of 5. Repeat 2 more times.

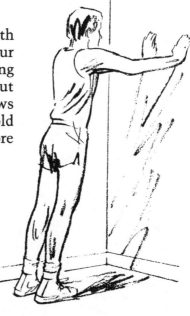

Warm-up Exercise #5:

Sitting with feet together, touch toes with head on knee. Then, stretch arms back above head and shoulders as far as you can. Hold for a count of 5. Repeat 2 more times.

Warm-up Exercise #6:

Jog slowly in place for a few seconds while moving arms forward and backward. The warm-up is now complete. Proceed to the general part of interval training.

Interval Training: General Part

For overweight persons and also for underweight with spot problems.

Any of the following exercises should be performed 4 times a week for 30-second intervals of high activity and 30 seconds of low activity. Check Table II (page 101) for the amount of time per session for your weight. Maintain a pulse rate of 130–140 beats per minute (or 65–70 beats per 30 seconds) during the general part. You can do all of one exercise or go from one exercise to another among those listed, but you must exercise for the correct amount of time. When switching exercises, be sure that you are not prolonging the rest periods more than 30 seconds.

Whether you are slim, slightly overweight, or obese, you must first practice one of the following aerobic exercises before going on to specific part exercises.

AEROBIC EXERCISES

Aerobic Exercise #1: Walking

If you don't know how physically fit you are, start your program with a low-intensity activity such as walking to avoid injuries. It is especially recommended for anybody over age fifty, those who are quite overweight, and people who have never exercised.

Slow walking is a pleasant activity but, unfortunately, it is of very little help in losing fat. Short bursts of fast walking should be alternated with short periods of slow walking. Two city blocks at a fast pace can be interspersed with strolling for one city block. Check your pulse to keep it at 130–140 beats per minute. Since walking is the least strenuous exercise, you can bend the rules a little and exceed the 9 minutes of activity a day. Thirty minutes of walking is enough to get results. Do it 4 times a week. Walking shoes should have low heels and soft soles; otherwise your legs will not pump blood efficiently and fat will not be burned. When your pulse fails to rise to the specified target after fast walking, it means that you are ready for walking/jogging.

Aerobic Exercise #2: Jogging

Jogging is a good aerobic exercise for general conditioning. It requires a higher level of activity than fast walking and is the natural transition from walking to running.

Walk slowly for 15 seconds, then jog for 30 seconds. You should walk/jog 4 times a week for a maximum exercise time of 9 minutes (see Table II, page 101). Wear running shoes, because jogging can be hard on your feet.

Let me set the record straight on jogging and fat loss. I'm not a jogging fan for several reasons. For the jogger who goes out for an hour in the morning, jogging mostly increases slow-twist cells; I'm trying to foster your fast-twist ones. And long-term jogging produces a constant pounding in your lower limbs that increases leg fluid congestion and decreases local fat breakdown. Finally, it is hard on your knees. Why, then, should you bother with it? Jogging is an easy, cheap way to obtain a general conditioning effect, and it is a good transitional exercise from walking to running.

Jogging does not improve your thighs, but it definitely helps in reducing big stomachs because it improves blood circulation in the abdominal region.

Aerobic Exercise #3: Running

The next level of interval training is walking/running. You should be physically fit to be at this level. After a warm-up, walk fast for 30 seconds, then run for 30 seconds, then go back to walking fast, and so on. Keep this intensity of exercise for the amount of time specified for your weight category on page 101. Do not exceed your pulse target. Run until moderately winded, then walk up to recovery even if you did not run for 30 seconds, and then run again. You can control your pulse by increasing or decreasing your walking speed.

Heavy sweating is a normal feature of walking/running. Sweat does not mean you are overdoing it. Your pulse is the only reliable indication of the intensity of your exercise.

Aerobic Exercise #4: Bicycling

Bicycling is one of the best exercises. It has several advantages over walking/jogging and jogging/running. First, it can be performed indoors, on a stationary bike, or outdoors. Second, your legs do not support weight, so anyone who is excessively overweight or suffering from knee or foot pain can do it. Third, there are reports that bicycling might help prevent and even improve arthritic knees. Fourth, with a stationary bicycle, resistance can be adjusted upward or downward. *Warning:* Do not ride on busy streets.

Adjust the bicycle seat as high as possible so that only the balls of your feet reach the pedals at the lowest position. Your leg should be fully extended with only the front part of the foot touching the pedal when in the lowest position. When working on a stationary bicycle, adjust the resistance so you feel as if you were pedaling up a slight slope. Pedaling with no resistance is not allowed. Work 30 seconds at a speed of approximately 30 pedal revolutions (1 revolution per second). Rest 30 seconds and work again. If your pulse does not rise to 130–140 after 2 minutes, increase the speed of your pedaling. Resistance should be increased when you are close to maximum pedaling speed and your pulse fails to rise. Pedal for the amount of time indicated for your weight on page 101.

Aerobic Exercise #5: Skipping Rope

Skipping rope is a convenient and inexpensive way of exercising to lose weight all over. When overweights are given a choice of different exercise techniques, skipping rope is preferred to running. Bicycling (perhaps because of the sitting position) is the overweight's favorite exercise technique. Skipping rope at the rate of 70–85 jumps per minute uses the large muscles of the body, activates fast-twist and slow-twist cells, and consumes lots of calories. Skipping rope can be a strenuous exercise, requiring 60–70 percent of your maximum work capacity. Overweights sometimes complain of tender knees and feet after a couple of sessions of jumping rope. Joint tenderness probably occurs because of the excessive weight that pounds their feet and knees 80 times a minute. Why bother with it, then?

After you have obtained the desired degree of fitness with four weeks of running, bicycling, or other aerobic activities, jumping rope is the easiest way to maintain your weight loss and fitness. You should not be more than 20 pounds overweight when you start skipping rope. If you have arthritis of the knees or gout, do not try this exercise.

Use a good-quality rope from a sporting goods store. Wear well-padded sneakers. Never jump rope bare-footed. Start with 30 seconds of activity followed by 30 seconds of rest. Check your pulse and keep it at your target of 130–140 beats per minute. When you become well trained, increase the time of your activity period to 45 seconds and decrease rest periods to 15 seconds.

You may use a weighted rope (½–1-pound weights at rope ends) to increase your arm exercise. During the first few sessions, jump at a leisurely pace to give your body time to adjust. Walk during the rest periods. When conditioned, you can increase the skipping rate.

Aerobic Exercise #6: The D-Squat

I have named this exercise the D-squat because you will draw an imaginary letter *D* with your hands while you move from squat to erect and back to squat.

I have modified an activity that was created for the crew of Skylab 3. The astronauts used a device called MK-1 to exercise their arms, trunk, and legs. The only things you will need to get the same results are two 1-to-2-pound dumbbells or a couple of large, unopened cans.

The astronauts used the squat exercise to increase muscle strength; you will increase oxygenation of muscles and fat as well as speed up your heart. The different results occur because the astronauts repeated the squat exercise slowly; you will work as fast as you can. They worked against the resistance provided by the MK-1 device. The resistance you will meet is the natural resistance of the body and the weight of the dumbbells or the cans.

The movement of your arms should be coordinated with your body position. In the squat position, your arms are down and your hands are holding the weights between your knees. In the standing position, your arms are fully extended as if reaching toward the sky. Do not squat too low. Adjust your squat with the help of a chair—when your buttocks are down, they should just touch the chair.

Begin by holding ½-pound weights in each hand or a 1-pound weight with both hands. Move quickly for 30 seconds from squat to standing and back while your arms simultaneously go close to your body from downward to upward, then, with arms straight, forward and downward again. Rest for 30 seconds. Keep pulse at 130–140 beats per minute. Stop when tired. Increase the weights when your pulse does not reach the target after 2 minutes of exercise. When you are trained, reduce the rest periods to 15 seconds. After several weeks of training you can skip the rest periods. You are fit if your pulse stays below 140 beats per minute after vigorous exercise.

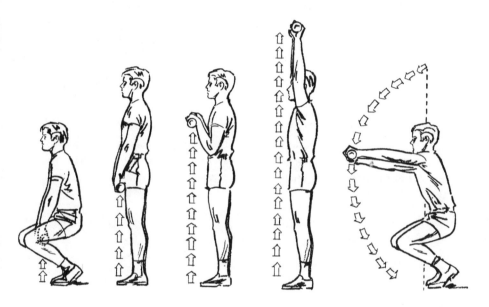

Interval Training: Specific Part

SPOT EXERCISES

The following exercises are for spot reducing. They should be done only after you have completed the aerobic general part exercises. Select the exercises that activate the muscles closest to your problem area. While practicing these exercises, your pulse will probably drop below 130 beats per minute. Raise it every 3 minutes with an aerobic activity such as running in place or practicing the D-squat. Most of the specific part exercises last only 1½ minutes, so you should do two different ones followed by a short aerobic activity. The total time for these specific part exercises depends on your weight and age. It ranges from 3 to 6 minutes and is added to the total exercise time. Check the table on page 101 for the ideal schedule for your weight category. If walking is your aerobic exercise, the total time expended on exercising can exceed 9 minutes.

Calves and Ankles

1. Stand up straight and rise up on your tiptoes. Hold on to a piece of furniture if necessary for balance. Return feet to flattened position. Do it fast. Work 30 seconds, rest 30 seconds. Do a total of 3 times.

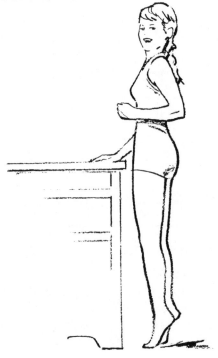

Exercise

2. Sit on a chair with your feet flat on the floor. Raise toes and balls of feet while keeping heels on the floor. Work fast—30 seconds on, 30 seconds off. Do a total of 3 times. If this exercise becomes too easy, add weights. You can use an ankle weight band fitted around the base of your toes.

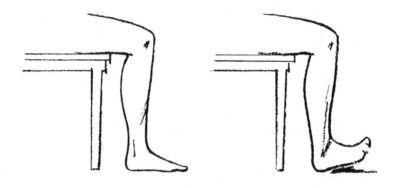

Thighs

1. To slim the front area of your thighs, sit on a chair. Begin without ankle weights in case you are unable to perform this exercise. Holding on to the chair, raise and lower both legs very fast—15 seconds work, 15 seconds rest. Do a total of 3 times. Tie 2-pound weights to each ankle when the exercise has become easy.

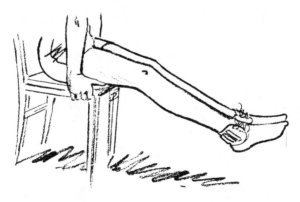

2. To slim lateral, front, and back parts of the thighs, attach 2-pound weights to each leg. Stand, holding on to a chair or table for balance. Raise the right leg to the side and return to the original position. Do it fast—15 seconds work, 15 seconds rest. Repeat 2 times. Swing the leg forward following the same routine, then backward with the same speed and periods of rest. Repeat 2 times in each direction. Keep leg straight in all directions. Before changing legs, raise your pulse by bicycling, running in place, or doing several D-squats. Change to the left and repeat the entire exercise.

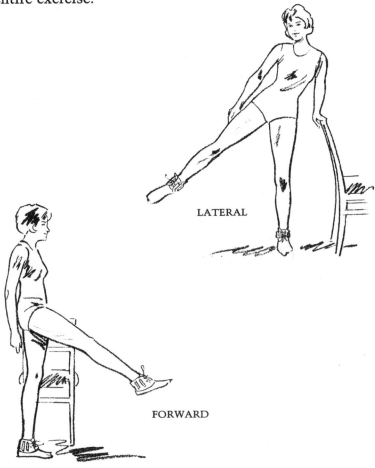

LATERAL

FORWARD

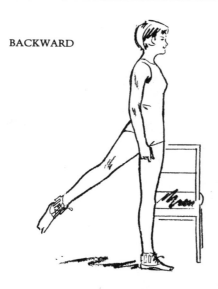

BACKWARD

3. To exercise the inner thighs and knees, sit on a chair and hold a pillow between your knees. Squeeze it with quick pressing movements of your knees. Keep your feet firmly on the floor a few inches apart. Quickly move your knees in and out. Work 15 seconds and rest 15 seconds. Repeat 2 times.

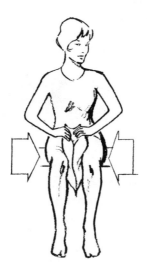

Buttocks and Thighs

From a standing position, do a half squat, then stand up again. Place a chair behind you. Your buttocks should barely touch the chair. Do the exercise fast—30 seconds activity, 30 seconds rest. Repeat 2 times. To increase the intensity of the exercise when it becomes easier, hold 2- or 3-pound weights in your hands.

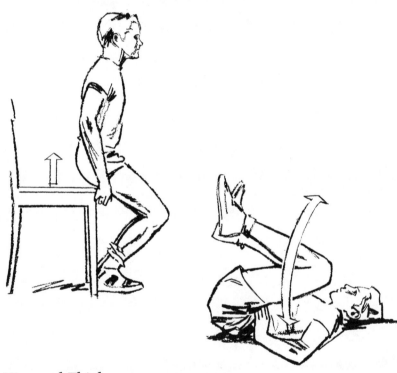

Hips and Thighs

Lie on your back on the floor with knees pulled up close to chest and hands on waist. Keeping shoulders flat and your knees together, rotate knees at moderate to fast pace in half circles clockwise and counterclockwise. Touch the floor with your knees on each side. Do 5 times in each direction. Rest and repeat entire exercise 3 times.

Exercise

Waist

Stand with the feet apart holding 2-pound weights in each hand. Keep your arms close to your sides. Bend to left side, then return to original position. Shoulders should face front. Do exercise quickly—15 seconds work, 15 seconds rest. Bend to left 3 times. Repeat the exercise to the right side 3 times.

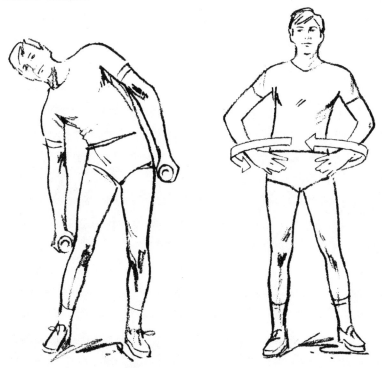

Waist, Abdomen, and Buttocks

Place hands at waist. Twist hips around in a horizontal circular motion while keeping feet and head steady. The pace should be slow to moderately fast: 15 seconds work, 15 seconds rest. Turn to the left, stop, turn to the right, stop, and turn to the left. Change direction after rest periods. Repeat 3 times.

Waist and Back

Stand with the feet apart and your hands clasped behind neck. Pull elbows back. Turn your upper body to the left as much as possible. Go back to starting position. Exercise at moderate speed—work 15 seconds and rest 15 seconds. Repeat 2 times. Now perform the exercise 3 times to the right side.

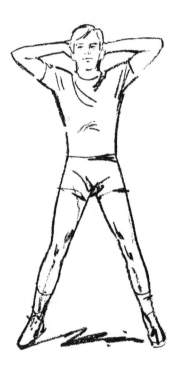
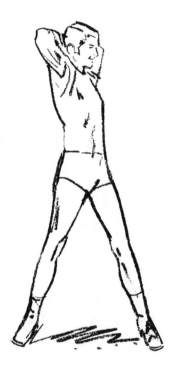

Abdomen

Lie on the floor, place your feet under a heavy piece of furniture, and bend your legs. Lift your torso slightly, then let yourself back down. Do not use your arms. You don't have to raise yourself all the way up—rise just enough to get your back off the floor. Do it fast—15 seconds work, 15 seconds rest. Repeat 4 more times.

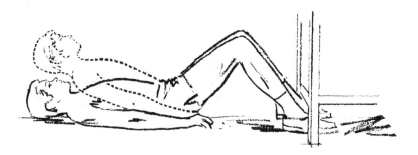

Arms and Shoulders

1. Stand straight with a 1-pound weight in each hand or on each wrist. Extend arms out. Make small circles with your hands. Do exercise fast—15 seconds work, 15 seconds rest. Repeat 3 times, then reverse the direction of circles 3 times.

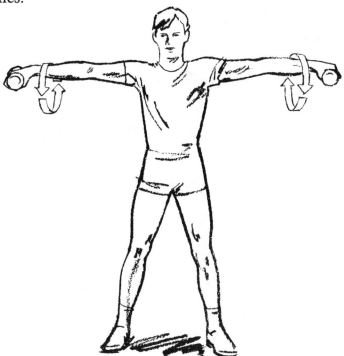

2. Hold a 1-pound can or dumbbell in each hand. Bend at hips. While keeping arms straight, raise and lower them quickly. Work 15 seconds and rest 15 seconds. Repeat 2 times. If you suffer from back pain, you can do the exercise without bending, but increase the weights to 2 pounds each and raise the arms just above the shoulders, like a bird flying.

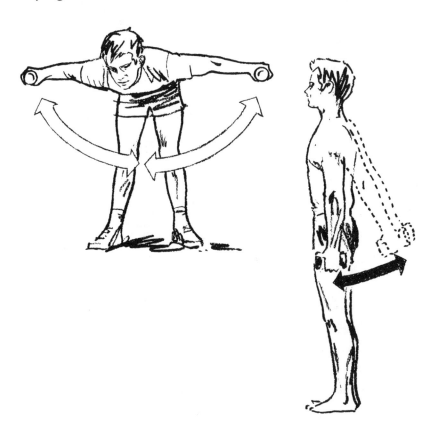

3. To trim the back part of the upper arm, hold a 1-pound weight in each hand. Stand with arms resting at your side, then bring them backward and up. Go as far as possible, then return to original position. Do it fast—15 seconds work, 15 seconds rest. Repeat 2 more times.

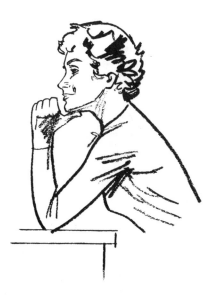

Chin

Rest your elbow on a table, then put your chin on your thumb and push down with chin. Do it quickly for 30 seconds. Rest briefly. Repeat exercise 2 more times.

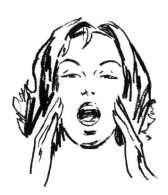

Face

Open your mouth and exaggerate saying *A, E, I, O, U* for 10 seconds work. Rest 10 seconds and repeat 3 more times. Lightly massage your face with the tips of your fingers while making the vowel sounds.

Breasts

Many women have soft and sagging breasts. There are no muscles in the breasts with the exception of a few elastic fibers at the nipples. Trying to harden the breasts by massage or the use of creams is useless. The only option is to prevent further deterioration by activity or diet.

Exercises help firm sagging breasts by providing strength to the muscles below them. They should be performed *slowly* for 7–15 repetitions. These exercises are not part of the interval training section; they are designed for sagging breasts only.

1. Lie on your back with the arms extended. Wrap a 2-pound ankle weight around each wrist. Keeping both arms straight, lift them approximately 15 inches off the floor. Return to the starting position. Repeat slowly 7–15 times.

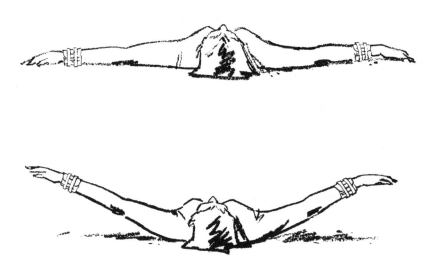

2. Hold a 2- or 3-pound weight in each hand. Bring your hands together at breast level, but do not rest hands on chest. Push one hand against the other as hard as you can, then relax. Keep weights at breast level and repeat 7–15 times.

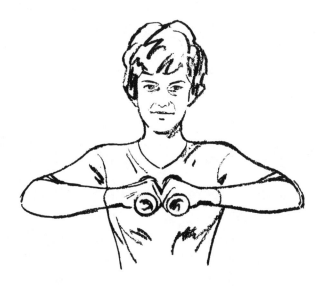

3. To decrease the size of the breasts, rapid movement is important. Do Breast Exercise #1 at a fast pace 7–15 times.

Special Situations

To stay slim you must carefully balance what you eat with the amount of exercise you perform. You might have to increase your exercise time or decrease the quantity of food you eat according to your daily weight. Weigh in daily and increase your exercise time if necessary. Do not stop exercising because you have lost enough weight! Weight can return very quickly. Specific part exercises alone won't keep you slim. You must keep up with the aerobic general part exercises. If exercise is not enough to keep you slim, you should start to diet again.

If you gain 2 pounds, do 2 extra minutes of interval training for a total of 11 minutes of general part exercises. If you gain 3 or more pounds, you should do 11 minutes of general part exercises and a week of the work diet. Keep records of your weight and exercise time.

THE TREATMENT FOR EXERCISE INJURIES IS "WEIRD"

If you start slowly, stretch, and do not overdo your exercises, it is highly unlikely that you will injure your joints or muscles. If something does go wrong, remember this acronym for treatment:

W(rapping)	Compression prevents swelling.
E(levation)	Keep the injured area up to minimize fluid collection.
I(ce)	Decreases possibility of internal bleeding.
R(est)	If you continue to exercise, things could get worse.
D(efer)	Postpone the next session until you have recovered from the injury.

A WORD OF CAUTION

You should have a physical examination before starting any exercise program. Your heart will be working harder, and screening will identify risk factors that could limit your program. If you are between thirty and forty years old, are healthy, and have no history of cardiovascular disease, the examination should include: a complete physical examination, an electrocardiogram (EKG), a urinalysis, and basic laboratory tests for CBC, glucose, cholesterol, and triglycerides.

If you are over forty, you should have the same thorough examination and your exercise program should be supervised. This is also true for people with diabetes mellitus, hypertension, arthritis, high cholesterol and triglycerides, hyperthyroidism, obstructive pulmonary disease, adrenal insufficiencies, renal or hepatic insufficiencies, angina pectoris, asthma, cardiac or vascular problems, detached retinas, or any acute or chronic illness, and for people who smoke heavily or are obese. A stress treadmill exercise test is recommended. Besides specific symptoms, you should watch for environmental conditions that would hamper or modify an exercise session, such as extremes of temperature, strong winds, high altitude, or a high pollution reading.

If you suffer dizziness, chest pains, or any unusual symptoms, stop the activity and call your doctor. Exercise can decrease blood pressure, and a hot shower, sauna, or steam bath can lower it further. Do not take a hot shower, sauna, or steam bath after exercising—you could become dizzy. Saunas or steam baths *before* exercise help warm you up and decrease the chances of injury.

Do not overexercise. Always work within your limits. Wear heavy, cushioned sneakers to protect your feet. Remember that you must exercise for the rest of your life. So go s-l-o-w-l-y!

Shoes and Leg Circulation

You probably wear shoes about sixteen hours a day. Shoes can have more effect on your lower limb circulation and fat structure than regular exercise. High-heeled shoes can undermine any exercise program because your calf and thigh muscles are kept in a constant light-intensity contraction. Long-term contractions strangle small vessels, tax the blood flow, and release lactic acid. Anyone with a tendency toward fat accumulation in the lower limbs should wear low-heeled shoes. When you wear high-heeled shoes, your muscles use only 20 percent of their capacity and burn tiny amounts of sugar fuel. This sugar fuel consumption, the increased lactic acid, and poor oxygenation all adversely affect the breakdown of fat.

Low-heeled shoes with soft soles such as moccasins allow muscles to pump blood throughout the limb. Walking then becomes an aerobic exercise because it increases the availability of oxygen. Excellent circulation and oxygenation are the first steps toward trimming fat.

Elevating the foot of your bed about 10 or 15 degrees can further improve return blood flow while you are asleep. It promotes venous drainage and decreases evening swelling. While lying flat in bed, exercise a few seconds to help venous drainage. Keep legs extended comfortably with toes pointed toward the ceiling. Point your feet backward and forward by bending at your ankles to undo daily high-heel miseries!

Massage, Steam Baths, and Saunas

Massage, steam baths, and saunas are pleasant amenities of gyms, health clubs, and beauty salons. They are useful in warming your muscles before exercising, and they contribute to cleansed skin and a feeling of relaxation. But are they helpful in losing fat?

Vibration and massage do not act directly on the fat cells. Their effect is mainly on local circulation. A massage releases substances that increase the size of the small blood vessels, so the blood flow to the area increases and more oxygen and other substances are exchanged between fat cells and the blood. Fat cells are not destroyed; they are just activated. The benefits of vibration or massage are short-lived.

Sweating is the major mechanism that the body uses to reduce the core temperature. Secretion of sweat can produce a body heat loss of up to 800 calories per hour. When your body temperature rises, as during exercise or sauna, sweating returns it to normal within an hour. Any weight loss produced by sweating as a consequence of external heat is short-lived; it returns as soon as you replenish the fluid you lost.

Saunas can be helpful in improving the metabolic activity in your fat. A recent study shows that saunas increase fat metabolic activity to twice the normal level. Whether this translates into more fat loss remains to be seen.

Cellulite

Cellulite is a diagnostic paradox. Cellulite is usually observed by a woman patient and denied by her doctor. Cellulite is so closely related to ordinary fat that most doctors dismiss it as a medical nuisance. This misunderstanding occurs because of the badly chosen name and its characteristics. The French word *cellulite* translates into English medical terms as *cellulitis*, a bacterial infection of the subcutaneous fat.

Cellulite is best described clinically as excessive fat deposits localized below the waist. There are areas of fat atrophy spaced between the adipose tissue which produce a dimpled surface.

In 1976, Dr. Willibald Von Kondziella associated the French term *cellulite* with a medical entity that was described in 1871 and called panniculosis. I prefer using the word *panniculosis* because it is free of semantic misunderstanding.

Treatment of panniculosis is difficult—to say the least. I have found that these atrophic areas cannot be modified, but excess fat can be removed by following my program. The end result is aesthetically acceptable because you reduce the fat mountains to the same level as the atrophic valleys.

How to Stay Motivated to Exercise

I have patients who would not exercise for a million dollars. If you are like that and unable to get started, try my imagery training technique to boost your morale.

Imagery training uses the imagination to improve your attitude and confidence. You mentally rehearse the exercise program several times before beginning to exercise. After the psychological preparation, the exercise program becomes surprisingly easier to perform. Be positive in the type and sequence of images. See yourself working with some effort but getting through it, finally ending the program a little tired but happy, treasuring your feeling of accomplishment. Repeat these thoughts a couple of times and then start the real thing.

Have you noticed how a tennis player who misses a shot immediately rehearses the correct movement to avoid missing the same hit in the future? Do as tennis players do and rehearse your exercise program to avoid repeating past mistakes. *Warning:* Mental exercise alone will not burn fat!

6
Relaxation Reflex

Tension and stress are common by-products of modern life. Chain smoking, nail biting, gum chewing, and excessive eating are external signs of stress. I am concerned with the stress effect on your eating habits. Overweight people often relieve stress with food, but I have developed a relaxation technique that will help anxious eaters to maintain control of their eating. Self-control is probably the most important aspect of sticking to a diet.

My technique centers on desensitization, conditioning, and relaxation. For patients coming to my office, I have prepared a relaxation reflex tape. You can order a copy by writing to Luis Guerra, M.D., P.O. Box 425, Planetarium Station, New York, NY 10024.

Or you can prepare your own relaxation tape. You will need a tape recorder and a 20-minute blank tape. A metronome is helpful but not absolutely necessary.

The first section of the tape should include annoying sounds that trigger anxiety. This is called "desensitization by challenging with stress," which means you become habituated to managing tension. The more you confront situations or sensations that increase your anxiety, the less you will react to them. You will be habituated to stress.

The second part of the tape is a conditioned reflex signal based on the Pavlovian technique. It marks the end of your stress and the beginning of relaxation. It is a sound such as a metronome, snapping your fingers, or repetition of a soothing phrase like "relax" or "be calm." Your body reacts to this sound or word as a signal to relax. When you have listened to the tape often enough, you will be able to calm yourself just by snapping your fingers or saying, "relax." You should use this relaxation signal whenever you are confronted with a stressful situation and before eating dinner.

The third part of the tape will contain relaxation instructions. You will learn how to contract and relax your muscles in a logical sequence to decrease tension in all parts of your body. This is followed by short breathing instructions and the hypnotic sound of a metronome.

Once you have recorded the tape, mastering relaxation will require 20 minutes of listening for 9 days. After you know the technique, you should replay the tape only once a week as a reminder. Muscle relaxation improves your health by decreasing your blood pressure, lowering your heart rate, helping you breathe more easily, and decreasing some unwanted chemicals in the blood. All of this has beneficial effects on neuroses, insomnia, and tension headaches, but most important is the fact that your emotional control will influence your reaction when confronted with food. You'll be able to control your emotions literally at the snap of your fingers.

How to Relax

There are several procedures to relieve tension. The simplest one is to avoid the stimulus that triggers it. For instance, if you hate to ride the subway, you can avoid that anxiety by taking the bus to work, and you'll get there in a better mood. But it is not always possible to avoid the situation that triggers an emotion, especially anxiety. Sometimes it is impossible to avoid a fight with your spouse. So you must learn a technique to control the anxiety that will result from a fight—you are going to be tense whether you fight or you avoid it by running away. This is known as the "fight or flight" response, which increases your level of tension regardless of the outcome.

The fight or flight response causes your muscles to

contract without your being aware of it. This is how your body shows that you are tense. You cannot directly decrease your internal tension, but awareness of the muscle contractions and the control of them have immediate beneficial emotional effects. Once you know your muscles are tense you can control this unwanted feeling. Control will induce a change in your body chemistry to regain your normal equilibrium. A preventive procedure for controlling tension is to contract and relax your muscles regularly on a daily basis whether you are tense or not. This will develop a critical awareness of the difference between the two states of being tense and being relaxed.

Desensitization

You should start the tape by recording sounds that annoy you most—a pneumatic hammer, punk music, a telephone busy signal, a dentist's drill, a baby's crying. If you are unable to capture enough nerve-wracking noises, you can buy a special effects record.

This part of your tape should last between 2 and 3 minutes according to your sensitivity to sound stress. If you have a short fuse, keep the challenging part to approximately 2 minutes. You can change this section of the tape by recording new annoying sounds when those already recorded no longer bother you.

Conditioned Reflex

The second part of the tape is a conditioned reflex signal that should last 60 seconds. It is a simple sound such as a tick-tock of a metronome or snapping your fingers at a speed of 45 sounds per minute. This signals that the tension is over and relaxation is to come. The reflex will occur only after you have listened to the full-length tape at least nine times. After that you will not need to listen to the tape to relax; you will be able to do so simply by murmuring, "relax, relax" or by snapping your fingers to produce a metronomelike sound.

You might remember that Pavlov's dogs were conditioned to salivate at the sound of a bell. Pavlov rang a bell every time a meal was given to the dogs, and soon the dogs salivated at just the sound of a bell without seeing any food. Human relaxation can also be conditioned by association. If a relaxation conditioned reflex is strongly conditioned to be triggered by a word or a sound, you will relax any time or anywhere without conscious effort.

Do not confuse the relaxation reflex with the aversion reflex used at some overweight clinics. The relaxation reflex is a positive reaction of well-being to a sound. Aversion conditioning pairs food with obnoxious words, images, or smells. Aversion therapy is a negative reflex of discomfort and has a very limited value. Punishment is always bad therapy.

Relaxation

The relaxation part of your tape consists of vocal instructions, which you will read starting on page 134. Read clearly and slowly in a monotonous tone of voice. The slashes (/) indicate a pause after each instruction, so you will be able to absorb it and have time to carry it out. Two slashes (//) should be a slightly longer pause. The technique you will be using is the Jacobson technique with some modifications.

The asterisk (*) indicates where the sound of the metronome begins. The sound of a metronome beating 45 times per minute is inherently relaxing. It is best to couple the rhythm of your words with the sound of the metronome: Re . . . lax/and be . . . calm" in a singsong manner. If you do not have a metronome, you can reproduce that effect by tapping a pencil on a table in a cadence of 45 beats per minute. To do this, you will also need a watch with a second hand.

Maintain a steady tone and don't speed up the instructions as you go along. Record in a quiet room, because any external noises will be picked up on the tape.

The relaxation part of the tape should take approximately 17 minutes. It might take more than an hour to record because you might have to redo it a couple of times.

How to Use the Tape

Sounds are not the only sensations that can be stressful. Another way to increase stress is to contract all your muscles while standing. Use your imagination to recall episodes of tension. You can start by imagining minor annoying things like the last parking ticket you got or the bill you must pay.

These complementary techniques are used while you are listening to the stress-challenging sounds of your tape. The object of all this intensive stimulation is to produce a high level of tension that lasts a short time and is followed by a signal that precedes pleasant relaxation. The higher your level of anxiety, the deeper your level of relaxation and the stronger your conditioned reflex will be.

As soon as the signal "relax" or "be calm" or the sound of fingers snapping comes on, dim the lights in the room, and sit down in a comfortable armchair. Softly murmur the signal word or snap your fingers following the rhythm of the signal. You can drink a small (4-ounce) glass of a cold, noncaloric fluid (iced tea, diet soda, water) that has already been set out. The tape will start the instructions for muscle relaxation, and you will follow them while in a relaxed frame of mind. All other activities should be discontinued when the muscle-relaxation instructions begin. Just enjoy the tape and follow the instructions.

The Tape

DESENSITIZATION (lasts approximately 2–3 minutes)

Record annoying sounds.

CONDITIONED REFLEX SIGNAL (lasts approximately 1 minute)

Read slowly in a natural tone of voice. Stress noise should be discontinued.

> VOICE: Snap your fingers or turn on a metronome at 45 beats per minute. Record the metronome beats or finger-snapping sound for about 10 seconds.
> VOICE: Slowly repeat "Re . . . lax, re . . . lax, be . . . calm, be . . . calm."
> VOICE: Now sit down in an armchair or lie on a bed. [Pause about 10 seconds before starting the next step.]

RELAXATION REFLEX (lasts approximately 14 minutes)

> / = 1 second pause   // = 4 seconds pause   * = metronome beat. Read very slowly in a calm, monotonous tone of voice.
>
> > VOICE: Stop snapping your fingers or end the metronome sound // Now, just settle back comfortably / You are going to tense and relax your body starting with your upper limbs / First, you will tense the muscles of your left hand, forearm, and arm by making a fist and flexing the forearm //

Relax these muscles slowly. Slow . . . ly stretch the limb, relax the muscles, let them go . . . until the arm drops heavily / Drops heavily // Now, tense the muscles of your right hand, forearm, and arm by making a fist and flexing the forearm // Gently, slow . . . ly relax these muscles, let the limb fall, let it drop heavily, let it drop heavily // Frown and crease your brow and wrinkle up your forehead now // Slowly release the tension of your forehead / Let go of all the tension // Now clench your jaw, bite your teeth together, and at the same time press your chin against your chest // Relax your jaw now, let your head return to a comfortable position, let it fall back, relaxing completely, relax all of these muscles / Let all the tension from these muscles go free // Now, tense the muscles of your shoulders, shrug your shoulders up, hold the tension // Drop your shoulders and feel the relaxation, let the relaxation spread deep into the shoulders, relaxing completely / Let the muscles become completely relaxed // Now, focus on your breathing, feel the air enter your nostrils and throat. Become aware of the rhythm of your breathing as your breath flows slow . . . ly in and out of your body. Take a very deep breath, hold it for about three seconds // Slowly release the air, relaxing your trunk muscles as you do so, relaxing them completely / Let yourself breathe gently, slow . . . ly, and regularly // Now tense the muscles of your left foot, leg, thigh, and hip // All right, let the limb fall slow . . . ly by relaxing all muscles, slowly releasing the tension until all the muscles in the limb are completely loose / Let the relaxation develop, spreading and growing deeper / Even deeper // Now, tense the muscles of your right foot, leg, thigh, and hip // Let the limb fall slow ... ly by relaxing all muscles, slowly releasing the tension until all the limb is completely loose // fully relaxed // Your body is now relaxed, let the relaxation spread deep into all the muscles, until they are free of tension // Feel the peaceful sensation that accompanies deep relaxation // ****Now, listen to the sound, listen to the sound // and / re ... lax, re ... lax // Let your body go free // Let your body go free // as you re ... lax your body goes free // re ... lax and go ... free // You begin to feel quite relaxed // All the muscles / of the body / are loose / All the muscles / of the body / are ... loose // You are feeling / heavy / and relaxed / Heavy / and relaxed // Your legs / and hips / are relaxed / and comfortable // Your arms / and shoulders / feel relaxed / and comfortable // Your neck / jaw / and forehead / feel relaxed / and comfortable // Your whole body / feels heavy / comfortable / and relaxed // In this deep state of body relaxation / your mind is filled / with calmness / and peacefulness // You are calm / and at peace / Calm / and at peace / Completely calm / and at peace / as you re ... lax more / and more / deeply / into mind-body relaxation // Your arms / and hands / are heavy / and warm / heavy / and warm // You feel quiet / and relaxed / while your body / is relaxed / and warm / A pleasant warmth // You are sinking / into an inward / quietness / and the more / you let go / the more / you relax // Deep / within your mind / you see / yourself / relaxed / and comfortable // Imagine that you are / on a boat / anchored by a quiet beach / it's sunny / and pleasantly / warm / sunny / and pleasantly / warm // You are on a boat / in a calm sea / in a calm sea / Calm / and relaxed / Calm / and relaxed // Waves / gently rock / your boat / gently / rock / your boat / as you re . . . lax your body goes free // It's a pleasant / relaxing / feeling // Body and mind are relaxed / Body and mind are relaxed // You're as calm / as the sea / Calm / as the sea // Quiet / and tranquil // Totally / relaxed / as you go / more and more / into total serenity / total serenity // Listen to the sound / listen to the sound // telling you / to relax / and be calm / relax / and be calm // Listen to the sound / listen to the sound // telling you / to relax / and be calm / relax / and be calm / as you go / deeper / and deeper / into total / serenity // A pleasantly / warm / and heavy / feeling / of peace // You feel warm / and heavy / a feeling / of peace / a feeling / of peace // Deeper / and deeper / into total serenity // Relax / and be calm / relax / and be calm // All / the muscles / of the body / are relaxed / and warm / Totally / relaxed / and warm / as you re . . . lax and go . . . free / re . . . lax and go . . . free / re . . . lax and go . . . free / To reach / total / serenity / just relax / and be calm / relax / and be calm / To reach / total / serenity / just / re . . . lax and be . . . calm / re . . . lax and be . . . calm / re . . . lax and be . . . calm // It's a pleasant / relaxing / feeling / A pleasant / relaxing / feeling / as you re . . . lax and be . . . calm / re . . . lax and be . . . calm / re . . . lax and be . . . calm // All / the muscles / are deeply / relaxed / and comfortable / relaxed / and comfortable / To reach / total /

serénity / júst / ré ... láx and bé caĺm / ré ... láx and bé ... caĺm / ré ... láx and gó ... frée / ré ... láx and gó ... frée

This should take approximately 15 minutes. If you did it in 10 minutes or less, do it again.

Afterword

Ideally, in order to lose weight, control of your body and the environment is necessary. Most of the time, control of the environment is not feasible, but body control is within your reach. The psychological and biological activities performed by your body influence food intake, absorption, metabolism, and excretion. You can modify all of those functions to accomplish your weight goal.

Food intake as a consequence of increased anxiety can be reduced by a psychological technique called the relaxation reflex. Excessive appetite produced by gastrointestinal hormonal imbalance can be controlled by specific type of food intake in a particular sequence.

Food absorption can be decreased by food constituents called soluble fiber and specifically by pectin. Metabolic activities can be improved by aerobic exercises and low salt intake.

Excretion is a result of the amount of food ingested, biological reactions, and gastrointestinal motility. The combination of a balanced intake of fiber and the improvement of motility produced by exercise will normalize this function.

The combination of Bio-Dieting, exercise, and relaxation reflex consistently performed for a three-month period gives you the best chance to make right your chemistry and stay slim forever. Many of my patients have done it; you can too!

Good luck to you.

Glossary

Adipose tissue. The body's storage area for fat.

Adrenaline. A hormone that activates the metabolic activity of fat cells.

Amino acids. The small components of proteins that are used by the cells in metabolic processes.

Arteriosclerosis. A degenerative process in the arteries that affects the heart, brain, and other organs and can lead to angina, heart attack, or stroke.

ATPase. An enzyme found in all cells of the body that pumps sodium out of the cells and potassium in to maintain the working levels of those substances.

Atrophic tissue. Tissue that is reduced in size and capabilities. Atrophic tissue is usually replaced by scar tissue.

Cholecystokinin (CCK). An intestinal hormone that sends the brain a message when satiety has been reached.

Cholesterol. A form of fat found in foods that is implicated in the development of arteriosclerosis.

Endorphines. Opiatelike hormones found naturally in the intestines and the brain.

Enzyme. The part of a cell that causes or speeds up a chemical reaction.

Fiber. A food constituent of fruits, vegetables, and cereals. There are two types of fiber: roughage and soluble.

Fructose. A simple carbohydrate sugar found primarily in fruits.

Galactose. A simple sugar.

Gastric inhibitory peptide (GIP). An intestinal hormone thought to increase the appetite.

Gastrin. An intestinal hormone affecting the appetite.

Glucagon. A hormone produced by the pancreas that opposes and balances insulin action.

Glucose. The body's form of sugar that is transported by the blood and consumed by the tissues.
Glycogen. A storage form of glucose.
HDL-C. A circulating form of fat that might protect the body against the development of arteriosclerosis.
Hormones. Chemical substances that are secreted into the blood or into the intestine in response to a stimulus, then travel to another part of the body to cause a response.
Hypothyroidism. Malfunctioning of the thyroid gland that produces slowed metabolic activity in most cells of the body.
Insulin. A pancreatic hormone that regulates sugar metabolism and has an important effect on protein and fat metabolism.
Ketones. Substances that are released by the incomplete breakdown of fats when the body is not consuming sufficient carbohydrates.
Lactose. Milk sugar.
Lipoprotein lipase (LPL). An enzyme that breaks down fat.
Metabolism. Chemical and physical processes constantly occurring in the body.
Neurotensin. An intestinal hormone.
Pectin. A soluble fiber found naturally in some fruits.
Secretin. A hormone affecting the appetite.
Serotonin. A chemical originating from the amino acid tryptophane that affects the appetite and mood by acting on the brain.
Soluble fiber. A food constituent that has the ability to decrease the absorption of fat, carbohydrates, and proteins.
Substance P. An intestinal hormone.
Sucrose. Common table sugar.
Triglyceride. The fatty acid that is absorbed and deposited in the body.
Tryptophane. An essential amino acid component of proteins.
T3. The most active part of hormones from the thyroid.

Index

Abdomen, exercises for, 115, 116
Adipose tissues (fatty deposits), 30–31
Adrenaline, 34–35, 94
Aerobic exercises, 18, 104–9, 122
  ATPase activity and, 20, 33
  bicycling, 106–7
  D-squats, 108–9
  jogging, 105
  running, 106
  serotonin and, 18, 21
  skipping rope, 107–8
  walking, 104–5
Age, metabolic rate and, 34
Alcoholic drinks, 79
American Cancer Society, 89
Amino acids, 14, 29
Animals, appetite in, 4
Ankles, exercise for, 110–11
Appetite. *See also* Hunger
  menstrual period and, 7
  senses and, 3–5
Appetite stimulators, 16, 21
Appetite suppressants, 16–18, 21. *See also* Apple pectin tablets; Safflower oil capsules
  fats as, 32
  tryptophane as, 37
Apple pectin tablets, 28, 37, 48, 72, 74
Arms, exercises for, 117–18
Arteriosclerosis, 82, 83
ATPase, 20, 33–35

Back, exercise for the, 116
Bicycling, 106–7
Bile, 14
Binges, 6–7, 74
  safflower oil capsules for controlling, 37
Bio-Diet, 21, 38, 41–85
  as appealing and tasty diet, 24–25
  break weeks, 42, 45–4, 54, 58–59, 62–63, 75
  fluids in, 46–47
  fruits in, 53
  the heart and, 82–83
  meats and other proteins in, 50–52
  No-Choice, 54–63
  spices, sauces, and dressings in, 52
  vegetables in, 48–50
  weekly weight loss in, 67
  work weeks, 42–45, 54–57, 60–61, 75
Bran, 27
Bread, 19–20, 75, 85
  toasting, 30
Breakfast, 8
  for break weeks, 45
  cereals for, 72
  as largest meal, 68
  peanut butter at, 74
  skipping, 77
  skipping some of the allowed foods at, 78
  for work weeks, 43–44
Break weeks, 42, 45–46, 54, 58–59, 62–63, 75
Breasts, exercise for, 120–21
Broiling meats, 29–30
Buttocks, exercise for, 115

Caffeine, 31
  metabolic rate and, 35
Cakes, 85
Calories, ATPase enzyme and, 34
Calves, exercise for, 110–11
Carbohydrates, 13–14, 22–25. *See also* Low-carbohydrate diets; Starches
  absorption of, 23–24
  in processed foods, 24
  soluble fiber and absorption of, 25–27
  thyroid activity and, 23
  water retention and, 36
Carrots, water-holding capacity of, 27
Cellulite, 125–26
Cereals, breakfast, 72
Cheese sandwiches, 75–76
Chef's salads, 68
Chewing gum, 7
Chin, exercise for, 119

143

Cholecystokinin (CCK), 16–19
  fat intake and, 70–71
Cholesterol
  absorption of, 27
  ideal level of, 82–83
  in shellfish, 80
Cigarettes, metabolic rate and, 35
Circulation
  exercise and, 90
  leg, 124
Citrus fruits. *See also* Juices
  pectin in, 28
Clinitemp, 94
Conditioned reflex in relaxation tape, 129–32, 134
Cookies, 85
Coronary heart disease, 82

Dancing, 79
Desensitization, relaxation and, 129, 131
Desserts, diet, 72
Dinner
  for break weeks, 46
  skipping some allowed foods at, 78
  for work weeks, 44–45
Dressings, 52
D-squats, 108–9

Eggs, protein in, 29
Endorphines, 15–16, 21
Exercise, 9, 89–126
  for the abdomen, 115, 116
  adrenaline and, 94
  aerobic. *See* Aerobic exercises
  for the arms and shoulders, 117–18
  for the back, 116
  benefits of, 89–90
  for the breasts, 120–21
  for the buttocks, 115
  for the calves and ankles, 110–11
  for the chin, 119
  emotional effects of, 90
  for the face, 119
  glycogen and, 24
  for the hips and thighs, 114
  imagery training before, 126
  injuries from, 122
  interval training, 96–98, 104
  metabolic rate and, 34–35
  muscle cells and, 90–92
  physical examination before starting, 123
  prescription for, 98–99
  saunas or steam baths before, 123–25
  for spot reducing, 93, 99–100, 109–21
  temperature and, 93
  for thighs, 111–14
  for the waist, 115–16
  warm-up, 101–4
  women and, 92–94
  yo-yo syndrome and, 95

Face, exercise for the, 119
Fast-twist cells, 90–92
Fat cells, 34
Fat distribution, sexual behavior and, 81
Fat intake, 32, 70–71
  proteins and, 30
Fats, 14
  CCK and, 17–18
  fluids with, 17–18, 21
  pectin and absorption of, 28
  soluble fiber and absorption of, 25, 26
  trimmed from meat and fowl, 76
  unsaturated, 32
Fatty acids, 14
Fatty deposits (adipose tissues), 30–31
Fever Scan, 94
Fiber. *See also* Roughage; Soluble fiber
  carbohydrate absorption and, 23
Fish, 30
Fluids. *See also* Juices; Water intake
  before meals, 43
  in Bio-Diet, 46–47
  CCK and, 18, 19, 21
  lists of, 47
  with proteins or fats, 17–18, 21
Food preparation methods, 54
Fructose, 22
Fruits
  in Bio-Diet, 53
  dried, 73–74
  as first dish, 43, 73
  home-cooked versus canned, 77
  pectin in, 27–28
  as second dish, 73
  sugar in, 22
Fruit starters, 53
Frying, 32

Gas, intestinal, 70
Gastric inhibitory peptide (GIP), 15, 21

Index

Gastric juices, 27
Gastrin, 16, 21, 27
Glucagon, 16, 18–19, 21, 27, 35
Glucose, 13–14, 22
Glycogen, 13–14, 24

Heart, 82–83
  exercise and, 89
High-density lipoprotein-C (HDL-C) levels, 82, 83
High-fat diets, 70–71
High-protein diets, 29, 70
Hips, exercise for, 114
Hormones, 15
  appetite in women and, 7
Hunger. See also Appetite
  during break weeks, 75
  as a chemical reaction, 9
Hypoglycemia, 5

Ice cream, 85
Imagery training, 126
Injuries from exercising, 122
Insulin, 14, 16, 18–20
  dramatic changes in level of, 19–20
  excessive, 31
  fructose and, 22
  hunger and, 9
  milk and, 23
  starch and, 23
Interval training, 96–98, 104
Intestinal gas, 70

Jogging, 105
Juices
  as appetite suppressants, 38, 43
  CCK and, 18, 21
  as snacks, 68

Ketones, 19
  morning hunger and, 35, 36

Lactic acid, 96, 97
Lactose, 13, 22
Leg circulation, 124
Lemon, 6
Lipoprotein lipase (LPL), 14, 31, 94
Liquid food. See Fluids
Liver, 14
Longevity, exercise and, 89
Low-carbohydrate diets, 23–24, 69
Lunch, 44
  for break weeks, 45
  skipping, 77
  skipping some allowed foods at, 78

Maintenance diets, yo-yo syndrome and, 95
Massage, 124–25
Meals. See also Breakfast; Dinner; Lunch
  first minutes of, 43
Meats
  in Bio-Diet, 50–52
  broiling, 29–30
Menopausal women, 81–82
Menstrual period, 7
  water retention and, 36–37
Metabolic rate, 33–35
Milk, 23, 73
Minerals, 14, 80
Morning satiation, 35–36
Motivation, 41
  yo-yo syndrome and, 95
Muscle cells, 90–92
Muscles, 33
  of women, 92–94

National Aeronautics and Space Administration (NASA), 95
Neurotensin, 16, 21, 27
No-Choice Bio-Diet, 54–63
Nutrients, 13–15
  pattern of intake of, 28
  U.S. Recommended Daily Allowances of, 74
Nuts, 29, 30, 76

Odors, appetite and, 3–4
Oils, 32
Olives, 76–77
Omelets, 68
Oxygen supply capacity, 96

Pancreatic enzymes, 14
Panniculosis, 126
Parties, 78–79
Pasta, 77
Pattern of intake of nutrients, 28
Peanut butter, 30, 74
Peanuts, 30
Pectin, 27–28
  pattern of intake of, 28
Pectin tablets. See Apple pectin tablets
Physical examination before starting exercise program, 123

Pizza, 85
Potassium, ATPase activity and, 20
Potatoes, 19–20
  cooking, 71
Poultry, 30
Preservatives in dried fruits, 74
Processed foods, carbohydrates in, 24
Protein, 14, 28–30. *See also* Amino acids; High-protein diets
  amounts of, 73
  in Bio-Diet, 50–52
  CCK and, 17–18
  complete, 29
  fat intake and, 30
  as first solid food of the day, 35–36
  fluids with, 17–18, 21
  as last dish of meals, 51
  soluble fiber and absorption of, 26
  starches with, 71

Rate of eating, 8–9
Relaxation, 9–10, 129–33
Relaxation reflex, 21
Relaxation reflex tape, 129–37
  how to use, 133–34
Rice, 19–20, 68
Roughage, 25. *See also* Soluble fiber
Running, 106

Safflower oil capsules, 37–38, 47, 68, 71, 74
Salt, 84–85
Sandwiches, 75–76
Satiation. *See also* Appetite suppressants
  morning, 35–36
Saturated fats, 32
Sauces, 52
Saunas, 123–25
Seasonings, 52, 71
Secretin, 16, 18, 21
Serotonin, 16, 18, 21, 90
Sex life, weight problem and, 81–82
Sexual hormones, 81, 82
Shellfish, 80
Shoes, 124
Shoulders, exercise for, 117–18
Skipping rope, 107–8
Skylab program, 95
Slow-twist cells, 90–91
Smell, appetite and sense of, 3–4
Snacks
  avoiding, 68

  bedtime, 72
  for break weeks, 45
  for work weeks, 44
Soda, diet, 6
Sodium, cellular, 34
Soluble fiber, 21, 25–28, 43, 70
  benefits of, 26
  pattern of intake of, 28
  pectin. *See* Pectin
Soups, 46
Spices, 52
Spot reducing, 93, 99–100, 109–21
Starches, 13, 23, 68
  method of cooking, 69
  proteins that can be eaten with, 71
  seasonings for, 71
  water retention and, 36
  when permitted, 69
Steam baths, 123–25
Stomach
  distention of, 8
  noises or pangs, 8–9
Stomach acid, CCK and, 18
Stress, 129. *See also* Relaxation
  endorphines and, 15
Substance P, 16
Sucrose (table sugar), 13, 22
Sugar. *See also* Sweets
  in fruits, 22
  soluble fiber and absorption of, 25–26
  visible and invisible, 24–25
  water retention and, 36
Sweating, 125
Sweets
  craving for, 5–7
  insulin level and, 19
Sweet tooth, curbing a, 6–7

Taste, sense of, 4
Temperature
  exercise and, 94
  of sweet solutions, 6
Thighs, exercise for, 111–14
Thyroid, 34
  carbohydrates and, 23
Thyroid hormones, 20
Toasting bread, 30
Touch, sense of, 4–5
Trace elements, 80
Triglycerides, 14, 82, 83
Tryptophane, 16, 18, 21, 37
T-3, 20

Index

Unsaturated fats, 32
Urea, 29
Uremia, 29
Urine, color of, 69
U.S. Recommended Daily Allowances (USRDA) of nutrients, 74

Vegetables, 21
   in Bio-Diet, 48–50
   as first dish, 43
   home-cooked versus canned, 77
   mixing, 49
   starter and filler, 48–50, 72, 73
Vitamin and mineral supplements, 80–81
Vitamins, 14

Walking, 104–5
Warm-up exercises, 101–4

Water as nutrient, 14–15
Water intake
   amount of, 69
   sweet intake and, 6
Water retention, 36
   pectin and, 27
Weather, metabolism and, 33
Weight, recommended, 100
Weight loss, rate of, 67
Weights, interval training with, 97–98
Women
   exercise and, 92–94
   menopausal, 81–82
Work weeks, 42–45, 54–57, 60–61, 75
Wynn, Victor, 82

Xylitol, 7

Yogurt, 73